Confronting Cancer

ISSUES

Volume 60

Editor

Craig Donnellan

First published by Independence
PO Box 295
Cambridge CB1 3XP
England

British Library Cataloguing in Publication Data
Confronting Cancer – (Issues Series)
I. Donnellan, Craig II. Series
616.9'94

ISBN 1 86168 230 1

Printed in Great Britain
The Burlington Press
Cambridge

Typeset by
Claire Boyd

Cover
The illustration on the front cover is by
Pumpkin House.

CONTENTS

Chapter One: Cancer

Chapter Two: Fighting Cancer

Introduction

Confronting Cancer is the sixtieth volume in the **Issues** series. The aim of this series is to offer up-to-date information about important issues in our world.

Confronting Cancer examines the current trends in cancer and its treatment.

The information comes from a wide variety of sources and includes:
Government reports and statistics
Newspaper reports and features
Magazine articles and surveys
Web site material
Literature from lobby groups
and charitable organisations.

It is hoped that, as you read about the many aspects of the issues explored in this book, you will critically evaluate the information presented. It is important that you decide whether you are being presented with facts or opinions. Does the writer give a biased or an unbiased report? If an opinion is being expressed, do you agree with the writer?

Confronting Cancer offers a useful starting-point for those who need convenient access to information about the many issues involved. However, it is only a starting-point. At the back of the book is a list of organisations which you may want to contact for further information.

*****

Cancer

Information from Marie Curie Cancer Care

What is cancer?

Our bodies are made up of groups of cells, each cell so tiny it is invisible to the naked eye. These cells reproduce themselves by dividing in a regular way so growth and repair of body tissues can take place.

Cancer develops when cells start to divide at the wrong time and in the wrong place, then continue to divide and invade nearby tissues and organs. It is this uncontrolled growth of cells that causes a swelling or tumour.

Tumours can be benign or malignant. A benign tumour is contained within a localised area and once treated doesn't usually cause any further problems.

A malignant tumour, however, can spread to nearby tissues and organs, travelling via the bloodstream or lymphatic system to other parts of the body where they may form new tumours.

These secondary cancers are known as metastases. It is because cancer cells move to vital organs such as lungs or the liver and prevent them working normally that cancer anywhere in the body is potentially life-threatening.

There are around 200 different types of cancer, depending on the cell type involved, and they vary greatly from each other and in the types of treatment needed.

How is it caused?

Cancer develops when normal cells start to behave in an uncontrolled way. The damage occurs to the DNA in the cell nucleus and when the damaged cell divides, its abnormal DNA is copied. The process can take many years. Available evidence suggests that over 70 per cent of all cancers which occur in this country are due to environmental factors involved in our lifestyle.

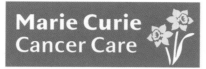

The most significant of these factors are diet, cigarette smoking, sexual and reproductive behaviour, alcohol and excessive exposure to sunlight. More than 70 per cent of cancers are therefore preventable.

What are the symptoms?

There is no such thing as a symptom that always means cancer. Because there are so many different types of

> *No one symptom means cancer. If something changes it is always advisable to speak to a doctor*

cancer there are an equally large number of symptoms. However, an early diagnosis of cancer is extremely important as the smaller the tumour when it is discovered, the smaller the chance that the cells have spread to other sites in the body, increasing the chances of successful treatment.

No one symptom means cancer. If something changes it is always advisable to speak to a doctor.

Some of the more common symptoms are listed below but it should be stressed that the most likely cause for any of these is not cancer – going to see a doctor is the best course of action.

- a persistent sore or ulcer on the mouth or skin
- a persistent hoarseness or cough
- a change in bowel habits – e.g. constipation
- a lump or swelling in the breast, or anywhere in the body
- persistent indigestion, vomiting or difficulty swallowing
- a change in a wart or mole – e.g. bleeding or increase in size

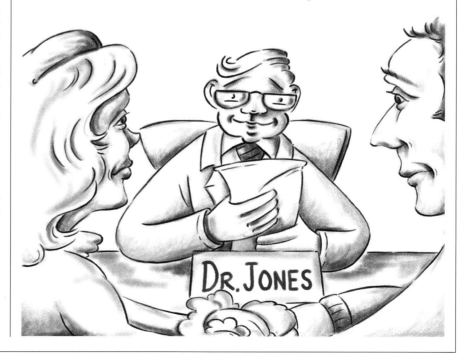

- bruising with no obvious cause
- pain or difficulty passing urine or blood in urine
- loss of weight for no apparent reason

How is cancer treated?

How cancer is treated very much depends on what type of cancer is diagnosed and the stage it is at; if it has spread and if it is confined to one organ or area.

In general, there are three types of treatment:

Surgery

Where possible, doctors will try to completely remove the tumour. It is important that all the cancer is removed which can sometimes mean a long operation, though not always. At some point during treatment most patients will have surgery – it is often important to establish the diagnosis.

The evidence that around 70 per cent of all cancers are caused by environmental factors is compelling.

Radiotherapy

Radiotherapy, the use of high energy rays to kill cancer cells in the part of the body affected, is given in one of two ways. External radiotherapy uses machines that produce x-rays or gamma rays which are directed at the cancer. Internal radiotherapy involves placing a radioactive source inside the body, which might be something like a tube inside a cavity, or inside fine needles inserted into the tumour area.

Chemotherapy

Chemotherapy is a whole body treatment. It involves drugs, called cytotoxic drugs, literally meaning cell poisons. The drugs circulate around the body in the bloodstream and can destroy cancer cells in different parts. Chemotherapy is given to destroy or control cancer cells which are known to be in the body though undetectable.

The top ten cancer killers in the UK

1. Lung
2. Bowel
3. Breast
4. Prostate
5. Stomach
6. Oesophagus
7. Pancreas
8. Bladder
9. Ovary
10. Non-Hodgkin's lymphoma

Can it be prevented?

The evidence that around 70 per cent of all cancers are caused by environmental factors is compelling. Although there are no guarantees, there are several measures which can be taken to reduce considerably the risks of getting certain types of cancer. They are:

- Don't smoke. As well as lung cancer, cigarette smoking is also responsible for many other cancer types as well as chronic bronchitis and coronary heart disease.
- Reduce the amount of animal fat in your diet.
- Eat more fibre in your diet – i.e. more fruit and vegetables and less meat.
- Be careful when sunbathing. Many types of skin cancer are due to sunlight, especially in fair-skinned people. Use a good sun screen – at least SPF 15.
- Observe workplace safety regulations – some industrial chemicals can cause cancer.

A cure for cancer

Modern cancer research – including research at the Marie Curie Research Institute – is focused on finding out which buttons to press.

The next generation of cancer treatments will be aimed at devising molecular tool-kits capable of fixing the damaged genes in cancer cells – particularly those that trigger cell suicide.

- The above information is from Marie Curie Cancer Care's web site which can be found at www.mariecurie.org.uk

© *Marie Curie Cancer Care*

Cancer is biggest killer

Cancer has become the main cause of death in both men and women according to new statistics published by the Department of Health. Between 1950 and 1999, deaths due to cancer rose from 15 to 27 per cent in men and from 16 to 23 per cent in women – overtaking heart disease, stroke and infectious diseases as the other major killers in England and Wales.

Yvette Cooper, Minister for Public Health, said: 'Cancer is now the biggest killer in this country. These new figures show how important it is that we have drawn up, for the first time, a national cancer plan, providing a comprehensive strategy for tackling this growing disease and reinforcing our commitment to improving cancer services.

'The plan is a major programme of action to link prevention, diagnosis, treatment, care and research. We know that the biggest reduction in deaths from cancer will be achieved through improved prevention measures, specifically a reduction in smoking.

'We have introduced a new target to reduce smoking rates among manual groups from 32% in 1998 to 26% by 2010 and we will tackle this by focusing on the 20 health authorities with the highest smoking rates.'

The latest figures on cancer trends, published in *Health Statistics Quarterly*, also show that people living in more deprived areas are at greater risk of developing and dying from ten of the major cancers.

If the number of cases and deaths from cancer were as low in all socio-economic groups as the most affluent, there would be 36,000 fewer cases and 26,000 fewer deaths from cancer every year.

© *Crown copyright*

Cancer statistics

Information from Cancer Research UK

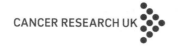

Introduction

Cancer is a disease that affects mainly older people, with 65 per cent of cases occurring in those over 65. As the average life expectancy in the UK has almost doubled since the mid nineteenth century the population at risk of cancer has grown. Death rates from other causes of death, such as heart disease, have fallen in recent years while deaths from cancer have remained relatively stable. The result is that 1 in 3 people will be diagnosed with cancer during their lifetime and 1 in 4 people will die from cancer.

There are over 200 different types of cancer but the four major types, lung, breast, prostate and colorectal, account for over half of all cases diagnosed.

Breast

Accounting for nearly 30 per cent of all new female cancers, this is by far the most common cancer in women. In men there are around 300 cases each year.

Lung

The most common cancer in men and the third most common in women, lung cancer with its low survival rates is the biggest cancer killer in the UK. On average 94 people die every day from lung cancer in the UK. The most important risk factor is smoking which, it is estimated, causes around 90 per cent of cases.

Prostate

This is currently the second most common cancer in men after lung cancer. However, while incidence for lung cancer is decreasing, it is increasing for prostate cancer.

Colorectal

Bowel cancer is the third most commonly diagnosed cancer in the UK and the second most common cause of cancer death. It predominantly affects older people.

Although cancer is largely a disease of old age, in many cases it is preventable. It is estimated that around $\frac{1}{3}$ of all cancers are caused by smoking and another $\frac{1}{3}$ by diet. Current government data report that around a quarter of adults smoke.

The incidence, survival and mortality information presented is based on population data. Survival rates, in particular, should not be used to make a prognosis for an individual patient for two reasons. Firstly, it is based on groups of patients with dissimilar stages of the disease and secondly, because of the need to follow up for 5 years, it may not reflect any recent advances made in the treatment of any particular cancer.

> *There are over 200 different types of cancer but the four major types, lung, breast, prostate and colorectal, account for over half of all cases diagnosed*

Cancer Research UK produce a series of CancerStats reports. Designed for health professionals, these include detailed statistics on cancer incidence, survival and mortality, and an overview of the latest information on risk factors, genetics, screening and treatment issues.

■ The above information is from Cancer Research UK's web site which can be found at www.cancerresearchuk.org

© Cancer Research UK

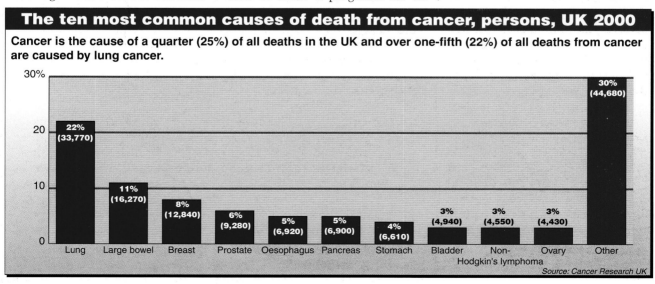

The ten most common causes of death from cancer, persons, UK 2000

Cancer is the cause of a quarter (25%) of all deaths in the UK and over one-fifth (22%) of all deaths from cancer are caused by lung cancer.

Cause	Percentage (number)
Lung	22% (33,770)
Large bowel	11% (16,270)
Breast	8% (12,840)
Prostate	6% (9,280)
Oesophagus	5% (6,920)
Pancreas	5% (6,900)
Stomach	4% (6,610)
Bladder	3% (4,940)
Non-Hodgkin's lymphoma	3% (4,550)
Ovary	3% (4,430)
Other	30% (44,680)

Source: Cancer Research UK

The 20 most common cancers

Breast

How many get it?
38,000-plus a year, 200 of them men. Taken over from lung cancer as No. 1 cancer.

Survival rate (at least five years): 74%

Who gets it? Mostly post-menopausal women, but 7,000 are under 50. Risk factor: family history

Treatment: Surgery (lump or breast removal), radiotherapy, hormone therapy or chemotherapy. Hormone therapy – tamoxifen – for 'oestrogen-receptor positive' types, meaning it is stimulated by the female hormone. Chemotherapy for 'oestrogen-receptor negative' types.

Lung

How many? Up to 38,000 a year.

Survival rate: 5%

Who? Smokers mainly. Most (24,000) are men.

Treatment? Surgery or radiotherapy for non-small cell types. Small cell cancer is fast-growing and can rarely be operated on as it has usually spread to other parts of body by time it's diagnosed. Chemotherapy is the main weapon against small-cell type.

Large bowel (colorectal)

How many? 34,000 a year.

Survival rate: 40%. Second biggest killer after lung cancer.

Who? Men are slightly more likely to get it than women. Risk factors: strong family history; poor diet.

Treatment: Surgery plus chemotherapy. Radiotherapy plus surgery for cancer of the rectum, but rarely for cancer of the bowel.

Prostate

How many? 21,000 a year. Second most common male cancer.

Survival rate: 50%

Who? Men aged over 60. Half of sufferers are over 75. Risk factors: family history; diet low in vegetables and high in animal fats.

Treatment: If cancer is small and slow-growing, it may be left untreated and just watched. Where larger but contained, prostate may be removed surgically or cancer destroyed with radiation. Hormone therapy may be used but side-effects include risk of impotence.

Bladder

How many? 12,500

Survival rate: 66%. Men have slightly higher survival rate.

Who? Seven out of ten are men, aged 50 to 80. Risk factors: smoking, certain industrial chemicals.

Treatment: Tumours removed by surgery, plus 'intravesical therapy': chemotherapy drugs or TB vaccine BCG applied via catheter. For invasive cancer: radiotherapy or surgery to remove all or part of bladder. Advanced: intensive chemotherapy.

Stomach

How many? 10,500 a year. Falling since Thirties, possibly due to better food storage and hygiene.

Survival rate: 10%

Who? More men than women. Risk factors: certain foods – high in salt, cured meats such as bacon or ham, barbecued and smoked food; alcohol; smoking.

Small cell cancer is fast-growing and can rarely be operated on as it has usually spread to other parts of body by time it's diagnosed

---

Treatment: Surgery to remove tumour and part of stomach, sometimes plus chemotherapy.

Lymphoma

How many? 8,000 Non-Hodgkin's a year; 1,200 Hodgkin's a year.

Survival rate: 50% Non-Hodgkin's; 90% Hodgkin's.

Who? People with lowered immunity such as those on anti-rejection drugs or sufferers of rheumatoid arthritis. Hodgkin's is a disease of the young and elderly.

Treatment: Non-Hodgkin's: chemotherapy and immunotherapy with sophisticated drug Rituximab. Hodgkin's: chemotherapy, radiotherapy, steroids, bone marrow or stem cell transplants.

Oesophagus

How many? 7,000 a year.

Survival rate: 6%

Who? Four men for every three women. Risk factors: smoking; drinking; poor diet.

Treatment: Surgery, often accompanied by chemotherapy. In advanced cases, chemotherapy alone. Radiotherapy can help prevent cancer returning.

Ovarian

How many? 7,000 a year. Fourth most common female cancer.

Survival rate: 30%

Who? Risk factors; family history; diet high in animal fat; using talcum powder intimately. Child-bearing and breast-feeding reduce chances of getting it.

Treatment: Removal of the ovaries and womb, plus chemotherapy using the drug carboplatin, or radiotherapy.

Pancreatic

How many? 6,500 a year.

Survival rate: 2%

Who? Middle-aged or elderly men and women. Risk factors: smoking; diet high in proteins but low in vegetables; history of diabetes or pancreatitis.

Treatment: Rarely diagnosed until advanced. Surgery to remove tumour or relieve symptoms, or radiotherapy to shrink tumour. Chemotherapy drug gemcitabine for those unable to have surgery.

Leukaemia

How many? 6,000 a year.

Survival rate: 33%.

Who? Most common childhood cancer, but affects far more adults. Half of all cases aged over 60. Risk factors: family history; exposure to chemicals such as benzene; possibly exposure to electromagnetic fields and radiation.

Treatment: Steroids and chemotherapy with the drug chlorambucil. Bone marrow and stem cell transplants. High-dose radiotherapy, chemotherapy.

Kidney

How many? 6,000 a year.

Survival rate: 40%.

Who? Twice as many men as women, mostly aged 40 to 80. Risk factors: obesity; smoking; well-cooked meat; exposure to certain chemicals; sometimes hereditary.

Treatment: Surgery. If not possible, 'arterial embolisation' – cutting off blood supply to tumour. Advanced cases treated with radiotherapy, chemotherapy and 'biological therapy' – treatment with a substance made naturally by the body, such as interferon alpha.

Melanoma (skin)

How many? 5,000 a year.

Survival rate: 80%.

Who? More women than men. Risk factors: ultra-violet light (sun or sunbeds); family history; moles; fair skin and blue eyes; burning easily; perhaps the Pill.

Treatment: Removal of affected mole. Advanced: chemotherapy, radiotherapy and immunotherapy. Drugs that stimulate body to react biologically.

Womb

How many? 4,800 a year.

Survival rate: 75%.

Who? Most common in women aged 50 to 70. Risk factors: overweight; high-fat diet; not having children.

Treatment: Slow-growing so often caught early. Surgery – hysterectomy – sometimes plus radiotherapy. Hormone therapy used to slow cancer growth.

Brain

How many? 4,000 a year.

Survival rate: 25%

Who? More common childhood cancer in under-12s; also over-40s. More men than women. Risk factors; impaired immune system; exposure of head to radiotherapy; contact wither certain chemicals.

Treatment: Steroids to relieve swelling plus surgery. Chemotherapy.

Mouth and lips

How many? About 4,000 a year.

Survival rate: Three in five. Lip cancer is easier to treat than other parts of the mouth.

Who? Smokers and drinkers.

Treatment: Surgery and radiotherapy.

Cervical

How many? 3,200 a year.

Survival rate: About 65 per cent.

Who? Risk factors include infection with genital warts, smoking, poor diet.

Treatment: It is important for women to have cervical smears to catch pre-cancerous cells as early as

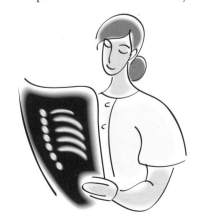

possible. Early cervical cancer can be cured with either surgery or radiotherapy. In advanced cancer, chemotherapy may increase survival rates.

Multiple myeloma

How many? 3,200 a year.

Survival rate: About one in four.

Who? Myeloma is a cancer that develops in plasma cells in bone marrow. As it is often found in more than one place – perhaps pelvis, spine and ribcage – it is called multiple myeloma. Risk increases with age. Twice as common in black people as white.

Treatment: Chemotherapy. Stem cell or bone marrow transplants may be tried.

Testicular

How many? 1,600 a year.

Survival rate: More than 90% cured.

Who? It is the most common cancer among young men. It particularly affects the 15-49 age group. Risk factors include family history and being an affluent white Caucasian. Having an undescended testicle can increase the risk tenfold.

Treatment: Removal of the affected testicle by surgery is the best treatment. This may be accompanied by radiotherapy or chemotherapy. So long as only one testicle is affected, the man should still be fertile.

Liver

How many? 1,500 a year.

Survival rate: Very poor, perhaps one in 50.

Who? Liver cancer should not be confused with secondary liver cancer, where it has spread from other parts of the body. Risks factors include alcohol abuse, hepatitis, cirrhosis, use of anabolic steroids, certain chemicals and, possibly smoking.

Treatment: Surgery is the main treatment when the cancer is confined to one part of the liver. Chemotherapy can help control the growth of the cancer if surgery is not possible. Radiotherapy may relieve symptoms.

© *The Daily Mail*
March, 2002

UK cancer survival rates 'worst in Europe'

Cancer sufferers in the UK have the worst survival record in the developed world, according to a major survey published today.

The study by market analysts Datamonitor found that British cancer patients were more likely to die than those in Europe or the US due to poor NHS funding, public awareness and screening programmes, which led to late diagnosis of the disease.

Oncology analyst Kyung Lee said: 'Low spending on healthcare expenditure by the UK government has significantly contributed to poor survival for cancer patients in the UK, rendering this rate amongst the lowest in the developed countries.

'The lack of funding has meant that not only is there low-level spending on cancer drugs and treatment facilities, but also insufficient cancer specialists who can provide best care for these patients.'

The Department of Health (DoH) has contested the findings, which it claims do not take account of recent investment in cancer care.

But the analysts criticised recent decisions made by the national institute for clinical excellence (Nice) to limit the availability of expensive cancer drugs on the NHS.

Mr Lee said: 'The problem of low survival rates of cancer patients in the UK is likely to be exacerbated by the lack of availability of effective drugs.'

Datamonitor found that the five-year survival rate for colorectal cancer, where patients diagnosed early have the best chance of survival, was lower in the UK than elsewhere.

The survival rate for patients diagnosed in the first stage of colorectal cancer was only 70% in the UK compared with 90% in the US and 80% in Germany.

In the case of the first stage of breast cancer, five-year survival in the UK was 78%, compared with 97% in the US and 93% in other EU countries.

The research also found that cancer patients in the UK were far more likely to be diagnosed when the disease was advanced and significantly harder to treat, reducing their chances of survival.

Only 50% of UK patients with colorectal cancer were diagnosed in early stages (stages one and two) compared with 63% in the US.

For prostate cancer, 58% of UK patients were diagnosed early, compared to 70% in the US.

Datamonitor blamed the lack of screening for cancers, other than cervical and breast cancer, for late diagnosis and warned it had 'potentially fatal' implications.

'Despite most cancers being preventable or even curable if caught early, lack of awareness and screening programmes have further compounded the problem of low survival and many cancer patients continue to be diagnosed or treated at a later stage when the possibility of success is greatly diminished,' Mr Lee said.

> *In the case of the first stage of breast cancer, five-year survival in the UK was 78%, compared with 97% in the US and 93% in other EU countries*

A DoH spokesman said: 'We know that survival rates for cancer patients diagnosed over a decade ago were lower in this country than for comparable European countries.

'That is why in September 2000 we published the NHS cancer plan which sets out a programme of action to improve cancer prevention, deduction, treatment and research.

'This has been supported by significant extra funding. By 2003-4 we will be making available an additional £570 million for NHS cancer services.

'Datamonitor's figures predate the cancer plan and the significant achievements we have made since its publication.

'For example, over 95% of patients referred by their GP with suspected cancer are being seen by a specialist within two weeks and the latest NHS figures show five-year cancer survival rates are rising by 1.2% for breast cancer, 5.6% for lung cancer and 2.6% for colon cancer.'

© *Guardian Newspapers Limited 2002*

Cancer survival

One- and five-year cancer survival rates are given in the table below for the three most common cancers in men and women. These account for around 50 per cent of all cancers in adults.

	No. of patients	One-year survival %	Five-year survival %
Men			
Lung	52,064	21.4	5.5
Prostate	46,010	84.2	59.8
Colon	21,287	66.3	43.5
Women			
Breast	78,780	92.6	75.9
Lung	27,119	21.8	5.5
Colon	22,003	64.0	43.3

Source: Cancer survival England, 1993-2000, ONS, Crown copyright

Common cancer myths

Cancer and older people

Myth 1. It is better not to know that you have cancer.

Many people are tempted to ignore worrying symptoms or signs such as a breast lump, because they do not want to know that they have cancer. There may be a subconscious feeling that if you ignore it for long enough it will go away. But this is not the case. Modern treatments mean that, usually, the earlier the cancer is diagnosed the more effective the treatment and the greater the chance of a cure.

Myth 2. There is no effective treatment for cancer.

You may have seen family members die from cancer in the past and this may have left you with the impression that cancer cannot be treated. This is no longer true as there are now very effective treatments available for most types of cancer. Some people can be completely cured of cancer, while in others treatment can be effective in slowing down the disease, or delaying it for many years. In the great majority of people, no matter how advanced the cancer at the time of diagnosis, treatment can improve symptoms and quality of life.

Myth 3. I am too old for cancer treatment.

You are never too old for any illness to be treated. Older people tend to have more than one medical condition and need more medicines, and these may interact with cancer treatments. Choosing the most suitable cancer treatment may be more difficult for your doctors, but it is not impossible.

Some people worry that their doctors will not want to 'waste' expensive treatments on them because of their age, and that they will miss out on the best treatments. However, everyone is entitled to receive effective treatments for all diseases, and doctors cannot restrict treatment because of your age. The National Service Framework for Older People, which guides doctors

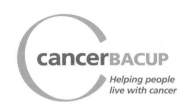

cancerBACUP
Helping people live with cancer

on their responsibilities and how to manage the diseases that are more common in elderly people, makes it clear that older people must have equal access to effective healthcare.

If you are not sure about the treatment that you have been offered, you can ask to be referred to another doctor for a second opinion. This happens very often and your GP can refer you to another specialist.

Myth 4. People with cancer always die a painful death.

Many people with cancer never have any pain, apart from the usual discomfort after an operation if this is needed to treat their cancer. If you do have pain, there are many pain medications available to help control it. There is no need for anyone to suffer uncontrolled pain.

Your doctors and nurses will work with you to control any pain that you do have, but it is important to be honest with them. Don't try to protect their feelings by pretending that they have helped you if you are still in pain.

Pain treatments do not become less effective if you take them regularly. It is better to take your pain tablets regularly, as your doctor has prescribed, to keep the pain away, than to wait until the pain returns and then try to get rid of it. It is better to take pain tablets, and be able to move around and enjoy a good quality of life, than to avoid taking painkillers and have to restrict your activities.

Myth 5. You can become addicted to morphine and other strong painkillers. Morphine treatment speeds up death.

People who need strong painkillers to control their pain do not become addicted to their medications, and they do not usually cause any harm. Sometimes, when you first start treatment with morphine or other strong painkillers, they will make you feel a bit sleepy and 'whoozy'. Usually this settles within a week, but if not talk to your doctor again. Other pain medications may suit you better.

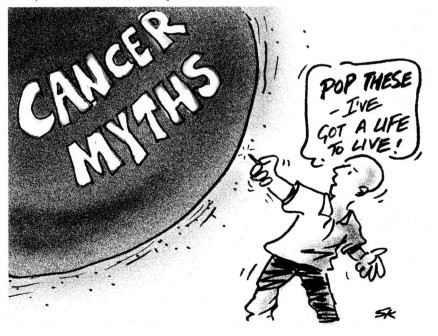

Most painkillers can cause constipation. If you become constipated ask your doctor for a laxative to keep your bowels opening regularly, ideally once a day. It really is an old wives' tale that morphine speeds up death. Many people take morphine treatments (e.g. MST tablets) for other types of pain (such as back or neck pain) for many years without any problems, and without it speeding up their death. There is really no reason to be afraid of pain treatments, or to avoid taking as much as is needed to control your pain and allow you to continue with as normal a lifestyle as possible.

Myth 6. Macmillan nurses only come to see you when you are about to die.

Macmillan nurses can be involved in a patient's care at any time during their illness. They may see a person with cancer soon after they are diagnosed if they have pain or symptoms which need to be controlled, or if they would like emotional support to help them cope with their cancer. Macmillan nurses are specialists in pain and symptom control, and in supporting people with cancer and their families.

Myth 7. People only go into hospices to die.

Some hospices work mainly through day centres, where people can attend for one or two days per week. Often they have home care teams, where doctors and nurses visit people in their own homes, to provide pain and symptom control and to give emotional support. Some hospices have beds for in-patients and these are often used for short stays, in order to get troublesome symptoms under control or to give carers a break and patients a change of scene. This is known as respite care.

This information has been produced in accordance with the National Service Framework for Older People, Department of Health, 2001.

■ The above information is from the CancerBACUP booklet series available from their web site: www.cancerbacup.org.uk
© CancerBACUP 2002

Children's cancers

Information from CancerBACUP

Children's cancers are rare. Only 1 in every 600 children under 15 years of age develops a cancer, and these are quite different from cancers affecting adults. They tend to occur in different parts of the body, they look different under the microscope and they respond differently to treatment. Cure rates for children are much higher than for most adult cancers and over 60% of all children can now be completely cured.

What causes cancer?
Nobody knows the cause of cancer, although there are many theories. A great deal of research is currently under way studying a number of possible causes. Sometimes 2 or 3 children develop cancer in the same school or village, causing local concern. These cases are carefully investigated but at present they do seem to arise by chance.

In general cancer occurs when cells in the body become out of control and multiply. They stop working properly and as their numbers increase they form a lump or *tumour*. When cancer cells break away and spread to other parts of the body they may produce secondary tumours known as metastases.

Cancers are not infectious, nor, for most cancers, is there any evidence that they are inherited. It is exceptionally rare for a second child in a family to develop cancer. Parents often worry that their child has a cancer because of something they did or did not do. This is not the case and parents should not feel guilty or take any sort of blame for their child developing cancer. Although the total number of children developing cancer has changed little in the last 40 years, the prospects for many have improved dramatically with advances in treatment.

■ The above information is from CancerBACUP's web site which can be found at www.cancerbacup.org.uk

© CancerBACUP 1999

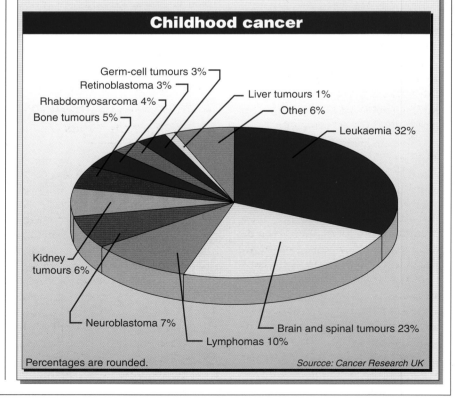

Childhood cancer

Germ-cell tumours 3%
Retinoblastoma 3%
Rhabdomyosarcoma 4%
Bone tumours 5%
Liver tumours 1%
Other 6%
Leukaemia 32%
Kidney tumours 6%
Neuroblastoma 7%
Lymphomas 10%
Brain and spinal tumours 23%

Percentages are rounded.   Sourcce: Cancer Research UK

Childhood cancer

Information from Cancer Index

About childhood cancer

Childhood cancer is rare, about 1 in every 600 children develop cancer before the age of 15 – still relatively little is known about its causes.[1] Childhood cancer is not a single disease – there are many different types. Compared with adult cancers they tend to have different histologies and occur in different sites of the body.[2] Common adult cancers such as lung, breast, colon, and stomach are extremely rare among children. On the other hand some types of cancer are almost exclusively found in children, especially *embryonal tumours* which arise from cells associated with the foetus, embryo, and developing body.

Leukaemia is the most common type of childhood cancer, representing about one-third of all cancers in under-15-year-olds. Leukaemia is a condition where too many under-developed white blood cells are found in the blood and bone marrow. Four-fifths of childhood leukaemias are acute lymphatic leukaemias (ALL), other types include acute myeloid leukaemia (AML) and chronic myeloid leukaemia (CML).

Brain tumours are the most common *solid tumours* in childhood, and make up about a fifth of all children's cancers. There are many different types of brain tumours: medulloblastoma, astrocytoma and brainstem glioma are the most common.

Neuroblastoma (sympathetic nervous system), retinoblastoma (eye), Wilms' tumour (kidneys), and hepatobalstoma (liver) are most usually found in infants or young children. Other malignancies found in children and young adults include lymphomas (Hodgkin's and Non-Hodgkin's Lymphoma), soft tissue sarcomas (including rhabdomyosarcoma), bone cancer (osteosarcoma and Ewing's sarcoma), plus a number of other less common childhood cancers. Histiocytocis is rare; it is not thought to be a true cancer, but in many respects behaves like one.

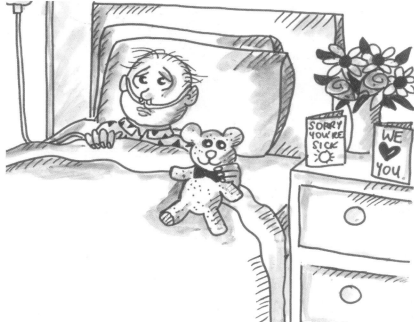

The cause of most cancers remains unknown. A minority of cancers are known to be hereditary (inherited). For example *some* retinoblastomas, and Wilms' tumours are thought to be hereditary. In rare cases the family may have a history of cancers (Li-Fraumeni Syndrome).[3] However most childhood cancers have no obvious hereditary cause.

> ### *Childhood cancer is not a single disease – there are many different types*

Children with cancer are generally treated by specialists. Medical professionals who have expertise in diagnosing and treating children with cancer include paediatric oncologists, pathologists, haematologists, radiotherapists, surgeons, radiographers, and others; all of whom work closely together, often in dedicated children's cancer centres. National and international children's cancer organisations have evolved in order to provide the best treatments, and are constantly engaged in research to further understand and develop better treatments for childhood cancer.

The overall cure rate for childhood cancer has drastically improved over the last 2 decades in association with clinical trials and the development of new treatments. [4, 5]

References

1 Stiller CA. Aetiology and epidemiology. In Plowman PN, Pinkerton CR, *Paediatric Oncology: Clinical practice and controversies.* Chapman and Hall Medical 1992.
2 Miller RW, Young JL, Novakovic PH. Childhood Cancer. *Cancer* 1994;75:395-405.
3 Birch JM. Li-Frameni Syndrome. *Eur. J. Cancer* 1994;30A:1935-41.
4 Lukens JN. Progress Resulting from Clinical Trials: Solid Tumours in Childhood Cancer. *Cancer* 1994;74:2710-8
5 Draper G, Kroll ME, Stiller C. Childhood Cancer. In: Trends in Cancer Incidence and Mortality. *Cancer Surveys* 1994;19,493-517.

■ The above information is from Cancer Index's web site which can be found at www.cancerindex.org

Young people are confused and want to know more

Two-thirds of children[1] know somebody affected by cancer, and nearly half have had a family member with the disease, yet they still lack understanding about cancer, its causes and their own relative risk. This is according to research published today by MORI for Macmillan Cancer Relief, to launch the charity's schools awareness programme Cancer Talk.

Accurate understanding of some facts is confused in children's minds by myths and unproven speculation which lead to unnecessary fear. For example, 88% correctly identify smoking as a key cause. However, many children[2] think that mobile phones also cause cancer (not proven), and 14% of 10- to 11-year-olds believe you can catch cancer from other people.

Three-quarters of children say that they would like to know more about cancer

---

Children also have mixed knowledge of the cancers which might affect their age groups. 19% rightly identify leukaemia as the type of cancer that young people are most at risk of developing. Yet nearly the same proportion mentions lung and skin cancers, even though these mainly affect older age groups.

Alarmingly, only 9% of the boys interviewed mention testicular cancer, which can affect males from 15 years of age, and is the most common form of cancer for young men. This form of cancer can easily be detected by self-examination and has a 90% cure rate if caught early.

One of the most significant findings from the report is that three-quarters of children say that they would like to know more about cancer.

Key findings include:

- One-fifth of young people see inheriting cancer from one or both parents as one of the ways people are most likely to develop the disease despite the low risk (5-10%[3]) of this happening.
- Only 10% are aware that young people are at risk of developing brain tumours, the second most prevalent form of cancer in this age group.[4]
- 82% of children state that more should be taught about cancer prevention in schools.
- Young people in the focus groups indicated that they would not feel confident enough about how to check themselves for any early signs of cancer, and rely on doctors to do it for them.
- Girls in the focus groups were more likely than boys to seek out information about cancer and follow up their questions – a trend which is known to continue into adulthood.
- Children in the focus groups mentioned that people with cancer can lose their social status, e.g. hair loss of cancer patients can lead to bullying in school.

References

1 aged 10-17
2 in the focus groups conducted
3 predisposition to cancer – source: Cancer Research UK
4 Childhood Cancers: 1 in 600 under-15s is diagnosed with cancer in the UK each year. There is a 70% cure rate. Leukaemia accounts for 430 cases each year and brain tumours 300, which together account for over half of all cases. Source: UK Childhood Cancer's Study Group/CancerBACUP

Note

MORI's Social Research Institute interviewed a representative sample of 437 young people aged 10-17 across Great Britain. Questions were asked as part of the MORI Omnibus, face-to-face in-home using CAPI (Computer Assisted Personal Interviewing). Fieldwork took place between 13-18 December 2001, 10-14 January 2002 and 7-13 February 2002. All data have been weighted to the profile of the population. MORI also conducted six focus groups with young people aged 11-16. Two took place in each of London, Edinburgh and Swansea.

© 2002 MORI

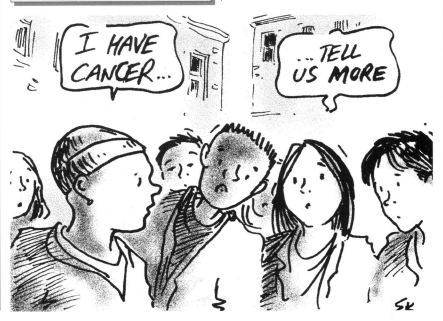

The challenge of cancer

The NHS Cancer Plan

One in four people in England will die of cancer. More than one in three people will develop cancer at some stage in their lives. Over 200,000 people are diagnosed each year with the disease – 600 new cases each day. Whichever way we present the statistics, it is not surprising that cancer is perhaps the disease that people fear most.

Progress so far

Over the past three decades progress has been made in reducing the impact of cancer:

- Overall, mortality rates are falling.
- Mortality rates for breast cancer have fallen by over 20% over the past decade – due to a combination of better treatment and the introduction of the national breast cancer screening programme.
- Falls in the rate of smoking among men since the early 1970s have led to a marked fall in the incidence and death rate from lung cancer.
- Overall, the number of people surviving more than five years has improved – an average of 4% every five years. These improvements are almost certainly due to a combination of earlier diagnosis and better treatment.
- Survival rates have improved dramatically for some cancers – especially for childhood cancers and testicular tumours. Almost two-thirds of children and over 90% of men with testicular tumours are now cured.
- Cervical cancer mortality rates have fallen by 7% a year since the introduction of the national cervical screening programme. This means 8000 lives were saved between 1988 and 1997.
- Hospice and specialist palliative care services (largely funded by charities) have been established across the country giving much needed support to patients with incurable disease and to their families.

The NHS has made progress in recent years in improving the organisation and delivery of cancer services. A comprehensive strategy on smoking is in place. There is strong support among health professionals for the strategy for cancer services set out in the Calman/ Hine Report and subsequent *Improving Outcomes* guidance, which are designed to spread best practice. And a new *NHS Prostate Cancer Programme* sets out new action and resources to deliver high class services and research for prostate cancer.

In the last three years the government has focused money and energy on driving up the quality of cancer services. Targeted resources totalling £80 million a year are being invested to improve standards and cut waiting times for cancer patients. And a total of well over £200 million is already being invested by the New Opportunities Fund and the government to modernise cancer equipment and improve access to palliative care.

Year on year the signs are that international medicine is slowly but surely extending its understanding of cancer and its capacity to treat it effectively. Many British medical researchers are playing a leading role in that work. Nearly a half of women and a third of men diagnosed now with cancer will live for at least five years and cancer survival rates are improving every year.

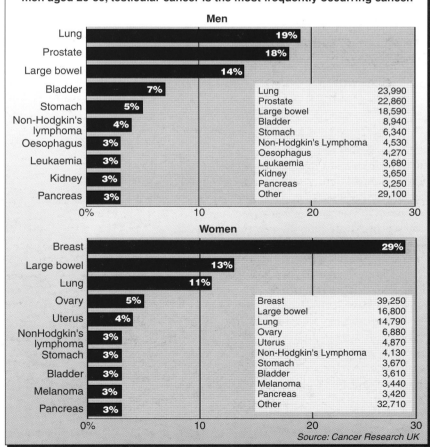

Cancer incidence

There are more than 200 different types of cancer, but four of them – lung, breast, large bowel (colorectal) and prostate – account for over half of all new cases. In the young, other cancers are more common. Leukaemia is the most common cancer in children representing one-third of all cases. In young men aged 20-39, testicular cancer is the most frequently occurring cancer.

Men

Cancer	%
Lung	19%
Prostate	18%
Large bowel	14%
Bladder	7%
Stomach	5%
Non-Hodgkin's lymphoma	4%
Oesophagus	3%
Leukaemia	3%
Kidney	3%
Pancreas	3%

Type	Cases
Lung	23,990
Prostate	22,860
Large bowel	18,590
Bladder	8,940
Stomach	6,340
Non-Hodgkin's Lymphoma	4,530
Oesophagus	4,270
Leukaemia	3,680
Kidney	3,650
Pancreas	3,250
Other	29,100

Women

Cancer	%
Breast	29%
Large bowel	13%
Lung	11%
Ovary	5%
Uterus	4%
NonHodgkin's lymphoma	3%
Stomach	3%
Bladder	3%
Melanoma	3%
Pancreas	3%

Type	Cases
Breast	39,250
Large bowel	16,800
Lung	14,790
Ovary	6,880
Uterus	4,870
Non-Hodgkin's Lymphoma	4,130
Stomach	3,670
Bladder	3,610
Melanoma	3,440
Pancreas	3,420
Other	32,710

Source: Cancer Research UK

But while other developed countries have broadly similar incidence of cancer, there is evidence to suggest that, for many cancers, survival rates for patients diagnosed a decade ago are lower in this country than in comparable European countries.

The reasons for poor survival rates

There are a number of reasons why cancer patients in England often have a poorer prognosis than those in other European countries. For some cancers, such as breast cancer and bowel cancer, this is partly because patients tend to have a more advanced stage of the disease by the time they are treated. This may be because they are not certain when to go to their GP about possible symptoms, because GPs, who see relatively few cases of cancer, may have difficulty identifying those at highest risk, or because of the time taken in hospitals to progress from the first appointment through diagnostic tests to treatment. Furthermore, the variation in quality and provision of services across the country means that not all patients are getting the optimal treatment for their particular condition.

Decades of under-investment in people and equipment have taken their toll. A service under pressure has struggled to adopt new ways of working and fully exploit new treatment methods to keep NHS cancer services at the forefront of international progress.

Equipment is out of date and is often incapable of delivering state of the art procedures for diagnosis and treatment. The NHS has too few cancer specialists of every type. For example, we have around 8 oncologists per million population, less than half that in other comparable European countries. And there has been a failure to modernise services by adopting new ways of treating patients. Incomplete standards of care for cancer services and inconsistent ways of assessing them has led to variations in quality of care.

Inequalities in cancer

There are wide inequalities in who gets cancer. People from deprived and less affluent backgrounds are more likely to get some types of cancer and overall are more likely to die from it once they have been diagnosed. In the early 1990s 17 professional men out of 100,000 would die of lung cancer, while the rate was 82 per 100,000 for unskilled workers.

There is evidence to suggest that, for many cancers, survival rates for patients diagnosed a decade ago are lower in this country than in comparable European countries

---

There are wide variations in cancer incidence and mortality related to birthplace. Mortality rates for lung cancer are lower in groups born in the Caribbean, Asia and Africa and are higher in people born in Scotland and Ireland, whereas deaths from cervical cancer are more common in women born in the Caribbean.

There are a number of reasons for these inequalities in cancer. While genetic factors may have some part in explaining ethnic variations in incidence of cancers, different levels of exposure to key risk factors for cancer – notably smoking and diet – are very important. The affluent are less likely to smoke and tend to have more fruit and vegetables in their diet. Lower awareness of the symptoms of cancer in some social groups, later presentation to GPs, lower uptake of screening services and unequal access to high quality services also play a role.

There are also inequalities in the treatment patients receive depending on their age. Not all patients are suitable for all treatments and it can be dangerous to give some very frail patients aggressive treatment with harmful side-effects. But frailty and age are not the same thing and some 70-year-olds are healthier than some 50-year-olds. As within any other disease treated by the health service, ageism is unacceptable in NHS cancer services.

■ The above information is from the *NHS Cancer Plan* published by the Department of Health. Visit the department's web site at www.doh.gov.uk

© Crown copyright

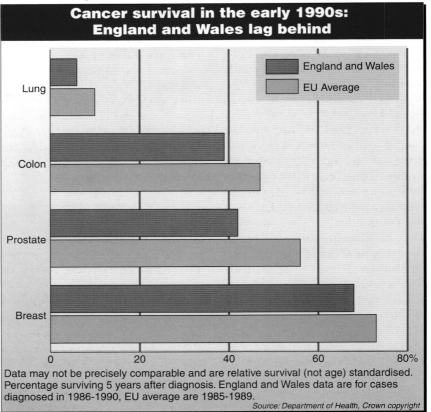

Cancer survival in the early 1990s: England and Wales lag behind

- England and Wales
- EU Average

Lung, Colon, Prostate, Breast

0 — 20 — 40 — 60 — 80%

Data may not be precisely comparable and are relative survival (not age) standardised. Percentage surviving 5 years after diagnosis. England and Wales data are for cases diagnosed in 1986-1990, EU average are 1985-1989.

Source: Department of Health, Crown copyright

Smoking and cancer

Information from ASH

Introduction

It is estimated that one in three people will develop cancer at some stage in their lives and that one in four will die from the disease. In 1995, there were 46,000 cancer deaths in the UK attributable to smoking: approximately a third of all cancer deaths. The UK Government has set a target (for England) to reduce the cancer death rate in people aged under 75 by 20% by 2010. The route to achieving this is set out in the *National Cancer Plan* which includes targets to reduce smoking. Cigarette smoking is an important cause of cancers of the lung, larynx (voice box), pharynx (throat), oesophagus, bladder, kidney and pancreas. A recent review by the International Agency for Research on Cancer found that, in addition to these cancers, smoking is a cause of cancer of the nasal cavities and nasal sinuses, stomach, liver, cervix and myeloid leukaemia.

Lung cancer

In 1999, 22% of all cancer deaths were of lung cancer, making it the most common form of cancer. Lung cancer is the cancer most commonly associated with smoking. Over 80% of all lung cancer deaths are caused by smoking. In 1999, 34,240 people in the UK died of lung cancer. Mortality from lung cancer in men fell from around 880 deaths per million population in 1990 to 628 in 1999, continuing the downward trend since the 1970s, which reflects the fall in tobacco consumption in the male population. Female mortality rates from lung cancer are still less than half the male rates: 301 deaths per million in 1999. This rate has remained stable throughout the 1990s.

One in two smokers dies prematurely: of these, nearly one in four will die of lung cancer. The risk of dying from lung cancer increases with the number of cigarettes smoked per day, although duration of

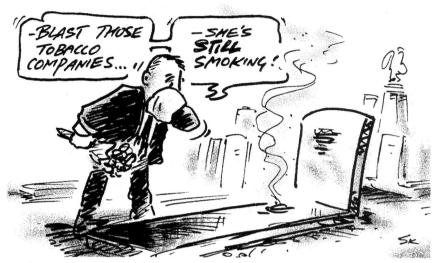

smoking is the strongest determinant of lung cancer in smokers. Smokers who start when they are young are at an increased risk of developing lung cancer. Results of a study of ex-smokers with lung cancer found that those who started smoking before age 15 had twice as many cell mutations as those who started after age 20.

A recent study by Peto and Doll examined the effects of prolonged cigarette smoking and prolonged cessation on mortality from lung cancer. They found that if people who have been smoking for many years stop, even well into middle age, they avoid most of their subsequent risk of lung cancer. Also, stopping smoking before middle age avoids more than 90% of the risk attributable to smoking.

Cancers of the mouth and throat

Smoking cigarettes, pipes and cigars is a risk factor for all cancers associated with the larynx, oral cavity and oesophagus. Over 90% of patients with oral cancer use tobacco by either smoking or chewing it. The risk for these cancers increases with the number of cigarettes smoked and those who smoke pipes or cigars experience a risk similar to that of cigarette smokers. In total, 3522 people in the UK suffered from oral

cancer in 1993. ('Oral cancer' includes cancers of the lip, tongue, mouth and throat.)

Heavy smokers have laryngeal cancer mortality risks 20 to 30 times greater than non-smokers. The risks associated with tobacco and alcohol multiply when exposures occur simultaneously: for those who both smoke and drink heavily, their habits are responsible for nine out of ten cases of laryngeal cancer in this category.

People who drink alcohol and smoke have a much higher risk of oral and pharyngeal (throat) cancers than those only using tobacco or alcohol. A US study revealed that among consumers of both products the risk of these cancers was increased more than 35-fold among those who smoked forty or more cigarettes a day and took more than four alcoholic drinks a day. It has been estimated that tobacco smoking and alcohol drinking account for about three-quarters of all oral and pharyngeal cancers.

Oesophageal cancer

Tobacco smoking is a cause of cancer of the oesophagus (gullet) and the risk increases with the number of cigarettes smoked and duration of smoking. The risk also remains elevated many years after smoking cessation.

Bladder and kidney cancers

Tobacco smoking is the principal preventable risk factor for bladder cancer which is estimated to cause up to half the cases in men and a third in women. As for lung cancer, the risk is associated with both the dose and duration of smoking, while cessation of smoking reduces the risk. Kidney cancer has consistently been found to be more common in smokers than in non-smokers and there is now sufficient evidence to show that smoking is a risk factor for the two principal types of kidney cancer.

Pancreatic cancer

Cancer of the pancreas is a rapidly fatal disease with a five-year survival rate of only 4%. Cigarette smoking is a strong and consistent predictor of pancreatic cancer although the risk diminishes to that of a non-smoker ten years, on average, after cessation. Risk of the disease is related to consumption and duration of smoking. A multi-centre study found that the relative risk rose to 2.7 in the highest intake category.

Stomach cancer

Studies have shown a consistent association between cigarette smoking and cancer of the stomach in both men and women. Risk increases with duration of smoking and number of cigarettes smoked, and decreases with increasing duration of successful quitting.

Liver cancer

Large case-control studies have demonstrated an association between smoking and risk of liver cancer. In many studies, the risk increases with duration of smoking or number of cigarettes smoked daily. Confounding from alcohol can be ruled out in the best case-control studies,

---

Smoking is a cause of cancer of the nasal cavities and nasal sinuses, stomach, liver, cervix and myeloid leukaemia

---

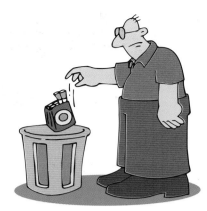

by means of careful adjustment for drinking habits. An association with smoking has also been demonstrated among non-drinkers. The IARC review concludes that 'there is now sufficient evidence to judge the association between tobacco smoking and liver cancer as causal'.

Colorectal cancer

According to the IARC review, there is some evidence that the risk of colorectal cancer is raised among tobacco smokers. However, it is not possible to conclude that smoking is a cause of colorectal cancer. This may be due to inadequate adjustment for confounding factors which could account for some of the small increase in risk that appears to be associated with smoking.

Cervical cancer

Cancer of the cervix has been found to be associated with cigarette smoking in many case-control studies. Until recently, scientists had been unable to decide whether the relationship was causal or due to confounding factors such as the number of sexual partners. A study in Sweden investigated whether environmental factors such as smoking, nutrition and oral contraceptive use were independent risk factors for cervical cancer and found that smoking was the second most significant environmental factor after human papilloma virus (HPV). The IARC review concludes that there is now sufficient evidence to establish a causal association of squamous-cell cervical carcinoma with smoking.

Leukaemia

A study of mortality among 248,000 US veterans of whom 723 died of leukaemia during 16 years of follow-up showed a significant increase in the risk of leukaemia associated with cigarette smoking, together with a dose response relationship between risk and the amount smoked. The risk was calculated to be 1.53 for current smokers and 1.39 for ex-cigarette smokers. A 26-year follow-up provided further evidence of a weak relationship between myeloid leukaemia and cigarette smoking in men.

Breast cancer

Some studies have demonstrated a link between both active and passive smoking and breast cancer. Seven of the eight published studies examining passive smoking and breast cancer suggest an increased risk of breast cancer associated with long-term passive smoke exposure among women who have never smoked. The IARC review concluded that most epidemiological studies have found no association between active smoking and breast cancer but since its publication a new study found that among women who had smoked for 40 years or longer the risk of breast cancer was 60% higher than that of women who had never smoked. Among those who smoked 20 cigarettes or more a day for 40 years, the risk rose to 83%.

Passive smoking

Non-smokers are at risk of contracting lung cancer from exposure to other people's smoke. The UK's Scientific Committee on Tobacco and Health found that the research findings were consistent with an increased risk of lung cancer in non-smokers of between 20% and 30%. This means that passive smoking causes several hundred lung cancer deaths in non-smokers each year in the UK. The IARC review confirmed that 'the evidence is sufficient to conclude that involuntary smoking is a cause of lung cancer in never smokers'.

■ The above information is an extract from a factsheet on ASH's web site. For a full list of references, see the full factsheet at www.ash.org.uk/html/factsheets/html/fact04.html

© ASH

WHO links passive smoking to cancers

By Sarah Boseley,
Health Editor

The government was yesterday criticised for failing to take action to ban smoking in enclosed public places, such as restaurants and offices, following an official declaration from the World Health Organisation that inhaling other people's smoke can cause cancer.

Yesterday a committee of the International Agency for Research on Cancer, an arm of the WHO, ruled that the scientific evidence on the carcinogenic effects of passive smoking was conclusive – something the tobacco industry has disputed for years.

'The group looked carefully at what non-smokers breathe in,' said Jonathan Samet, professor of epidemiology at Johns Hopkins University in the US, who chaired the committee. 'They are breathing in the same carcinogens as active smokers. Of course the concentrations are not as high, but they are breathing in carcinogens. They are being absorbed into the body and can even be measured in urine.'

The IARC committee evaluated more than 50 studies, involving more than 5,500 people with lung cancer, to produce their monograph – an official publication which they expect to influence the policy of governments.

The last monograph, in 1986, expressed the fear that second-hand tobacco smoke might be carcinogenic, but without evidence.

Although 90% of the world's 1.2 million cases of lung cancer every year are caused by smoking, tobacco is now thought to increase the risk of developing many other kinds of cancer as well

'This is the first time that IARC has reached this conclusion. To my knowledge it is the first time that an organisation with global sweep has reached this conclusion,' said Professor Samet.

There was considerable concern for children exposed to their parents' smoke at home over many years but, said Professor Samet, there was not enough data to determine whether they were at greater risk of developing childhood cancers or adult cancers in later life as a result.

Although 90% of the world's 1.2 million cases of lung cancer every year are caused by smoking, tobacco is now thought to increase the risk of developing many other kinds of cancer as well. It has been established that smoking is a factor in cancers of the oral cavity, larynx, oesophagus, pancreas and bladder. In some, such as oesophageal cancer, it is made worse by combination with alcohol.

Yesterday the IARC committee added five more to the list. According to its monograph, smoking is now proven also to be a potential cause of cancers of the stomach, liver, cervix, kidney and of myeloid leukaemia.

Sir Richard Doll, the veteran Oxford epidemiologist, said he felt strongly that cigarette advertising should have been banned in Britain. 'The promotion of tobacco I personally regard as something quite evil and the fact that it has not been stopped in this country I think is a disgrace.'

© Guardian Newspapers Limited 2002

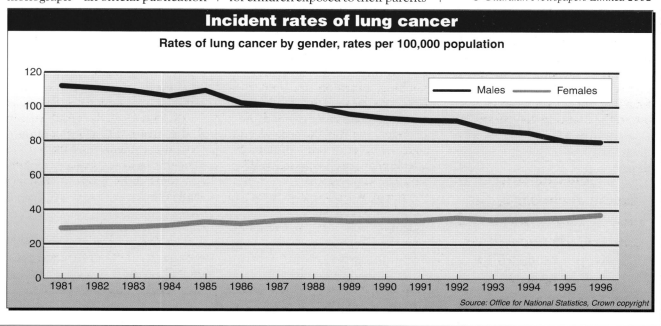

Incident rates of lung cancer

Rates of lung cancer by gender, rates per 100,000 population

Source: Office for National Statistics, Crown copyright

Body awareness

Reducing your risk

CANCER RESEARCH UK

Body awareness is all about knowing your own body and what is normal for you. There are certain changes you can look out for that could be early warnings of some types of cancer. Most of the time there will be nothing to worry about. But by taking action early and seeking the advice of a doctor, you could have a much better chance of being treated successfully if cancer is present.

Carrying out checks from time to time for changes in the way your body looks and feels can help to detect breast cancer, testicular cancer and skin cancer at an early stage.

Be breast aware

Breasts change in size and shape during the monthly menstrual cycle and at different times in a woman's life. It's important to get to know what your breasts feel like at different times of the month. That way you are more likely to spot an unusual change. Things to look out for are:

- changes in the outline or shape of the breast
- any puckering or dimpling of the skin
- discomfort or pain in one breast, especially if it's new and persists
- lumps or bumpy areas in the breast or armpit that are different from the same area in the other breast or armpit
- nipple discharge that is not milky, bleeding or sore areas that do not heal, and changes in the nipple position or rashes.

There are many reasons for changes in the breast and most of them are harmless. But it's important that they are checked out by a doctor because they could be the first sign of cancer. If you're aware of any changes in your breast, tell your doctor without delay.

Testicular cancer: it's a whole new ball game

Men should check their testicles from puberty onwards to establish what

feels normal for them. Although testicular cancer is rare, it is the most common cancer in men aged 20 to 39. The good news is that testicular cancer is almost always successfully treated, but detecting it early is very important.

The best time to check your testicles is in the bath or shower or just afterwards because the muscles in the scrotum (the sack that holds the testicles) are more relaxed.

Hold your scrotum in your hands so you can feel the size and weight of each testicle. It's quite normal to have one larger than the other or hanging lower than the other, but they should be about the same weight.

Next, feel each testicle and roll it between your thumb and finger. It should feel smooth. You'll feel a soft tube towards the back of each testicle, which is normal. This tube is called the epididymus.

Testicular cancer usually appears in only one testicle. Look out for the following warning signs

- a hard lump on the front or side of the testicle
- swelling or enlargement of the testicle
- pain or discomfort in the testicle or scrotum
- an unusual difference between one testicle and the other
- a heavy or dragging feeling in the scrotum
- a dull ache in the lower stomach, groin or scrotum.

If you notice any of these changes, see your doctor as soon as you can.

Malignant melanoma – be a molewatcher for life

The most serious skin cancer is called malignant melanoma. It often shows

itself by a change in the normal look or feel of a mole on the skin. If you notice any changes it's important to act straight away. Most changes won't be cancer but must not be ignored. Successfully treating malignant melanoma relies on catching it at an early stage.

You should be aware of the normal appearance of your skin and know where any moles are and what they look like. That way you'll be able to spot any abnormal changes or the appearance of new moles.

Most moles remain harmless throughout a person's lifetime. But some can start growing or changing their shape, which is a sign that a cancer could be developing. The most common sites for malignant melanoma are the legs in women and the back in men. In older people, the face is also a common site. But malignant melanoma can grow anywhere, even on areas of the body that are not exposed to the sun like the soles of the feet or the buttocks. Look out for the following signs

- an existing mole or dark patch that is getting larger
- a new mole that is growing
- a mole with a ragged outline – normal moles have a smooth, regular shape
- a mole that has a mixture of different shades of brown and black – a normal mole is all one shade
- an inflamed mole or one with a reddish edge
- a mole that is bleeding, oozing or crusting
- a mole that is bigger than all your other moles
- a mole that is itching

If you find a mole that has any of these features, see your doctor as soon as possible.

- The above information is from Cancer Research UK's web site which can be found at www.cancerresearchuk.org

© Cancer Research UK

Skin cancer deaths soaring as we soak up the sun

Britons going abroad ignore over-exposure warnings

By James Chapman, Science Correspondent

Holidaymakers were last night given a stark warning to stay out of the sun or face a hugely increased risk of skin cancer.

Some of the country's most eminent scientists warned that the British habit of sunbathing for hours at a time is beginning to take an appalling toll in lives.

Deaths from the worst form of skin cancer have more than trebled over the past 40 years because people are oblivious to the dangers, they said.

Figures released yesterday showed there are now 1,550 deaths each year in England and Wales from melanoma, compared with only 400 in the 1960s.

Even high-altitude winter sports holidays can expose the skin to high levels of harmful ultraviolet rays, because snow reflects radiation.

Scientists from the Government's radiation watchdog body also believe damage caused by UV radiation from over-exposure to the sun causes cataracts and other eye damage.

They said warnings about the dangers should be given on board aircraft heading to sunny destinations.

Sir Richard Doll, chairman of the National Radiological Protection Board – the scientist who discovered the link between smoking and lung cancer – chaired the NRPB's first review into scientific evidence on the damaging effects of UV radiation since 1995.

He said last night: 'Sunshine holidays abroad are, I'm sure, the main cause of the increase.'

Ad he warned against relying too heavily on sunscreens to protect against burning, adding that many travellers seem to regard them as an excuse to lie in the sun all day.

The NRPB report shows that skin cancers account for about 1.4 per cent of all cancer deaths in the UK. Eighty per cent are caused by melanoma, the most aggressive form of skin cancer.

The rest are caused by squamous cell carcinoma – which affects 7,200 people in Britain every year and kills about 440 – and basal cell carcinoma which is diagnosed in nearly 29,000 people a year.

The report adds there is overwhelming evidence that UV exposure causes skin cancer, sunburn, skin ageing and cataracts.

UV is also implicated in macular degeneration, an incurable eye disorder that affects two million people in the UK and is the leading cause of blindness.

The experts also condemned the use of sunbeds and tanning lamps, which expose the skin to intense bursts of radiation.

Professor Anthony Swerdlow, of the Institute of Cancer in Sutton, Surrey, who chaired the NRPB's expert group, said: 'Sunbeds involve an intense, intermittent, deliberate exposure of parts of the body that are not normally exposed. That is exactly the type of exposure that causes melanoma.

'Experts agree that the rising rates of skin and eye disease are due to sun exposure and the increase is large.

'In Scotland, new cases of melanoma have quadrupled since the 1960s, and there has been a similar increase in England and Wales.'

There is particular concern over the effects of sun exposure on children, he added.

It is up to parents to ensure that youngsters are covered up with hats and protective clothing, and use sunscreens, said the professor.

The scientists repeated warnings that fair-skinned people and those with large numbers of moles are most at risk.

Peter Lapsley, chief executive of the Skin Care Campaign, said: 'Greater exposure to UV radiation early in life can lead to an increased risk of melanoma in adulthood.'

© *The Daily Mail, February 2002*

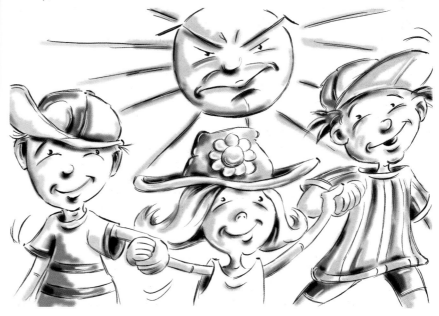

Sunsense

Protecting yourself from ultraviolet radiation

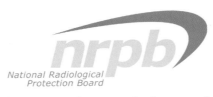

National Radiological Protection Board

Where does UVR come from?

Ultraviolet radiation (UVR) is produced by the sun and by some artificial sources. The human eye cannot see it. Two types of UVR from the sun reach the earth's surface. These are UVB and the less energetic UVA. Some people are also exposed to UVR at work, as a medical treatment or by using sunbeds.

Is UVR harmful?

The main source of human exposure to UVR is the sun. UVR can damage DNA in cells on the surface of the body. UVR causes the skin to burn. The skin may react to UVR exposure by tanning. It can increase the risk of developing skin cancer (melanoma, squamous cell skin cancer and basal cell cancer). Intense UVR exposure can inflame the eyes. Long-term exposure may cause cataracts. These effects can take many years to develop so over-exposure now may increase risks in later life. UVR causes skin ageing and, in many people, troublesome photosensitivity rashes. It may also affect the immune system in the skin, although the consequences of this are not certain yet. The incidence of skin cancer is rising. There are now about 40,000 new cases and nearly 2,000 deaths from skin cancer in the UK each year.

Surely, sunlight can be beneficial to health too?

Exposing the skin to UVR produces vitamin D. This benefit only needs the amount of outdoor exposure people get as part of daily life. It may be more important for health in dark-skinned people with vitamin D deficient diets. Many people 'feel better' out in the sunshine. You can keep these benefits of sunshine without increasing the health risks by following our Sunsense Guide below.

Are some types of UVR less harmful?

We do know that UVB is the main cause of sunburn. UVA is thought to cause skin ageing. We do not yet know enough to say which types of UVR cause cancer. The International Agency for Research on Cancer, which is part of the World Health Organization, classifies all UVR as carcinogenic (cancer-causing) to experimental animals.

Is sunburn dangerous?

Although there is limited evidence whether sunburn directly causes

---

Know your skin type

Which of the following best describes your skin's reaction to sun exposure?

- White skin that always sunburns easily, never or minimally suntans
- White skin that sunburns and suntans moderately
- White skin that sunburns minimally and suntans easily to a mid-brown colour
- Brown skin that rarely sun-burns and suntans well
- Dark brown or black skin that almost never sunburns

---

cancer, sunburn is a sign that the skin has been damaged. Your risk of melanoma (the main cause of death from skin cancer) is related, among other things, to the number of times you have had intense exposure to UVR. Such exposures may be particularly damaging in children, although skin cancers usually develop in adult life.

I have a suntan, does that protect me?

A suntan is a sign that the skin has already been exposed to UVR and is trying to protect itself from further harm. People with naturally dark or tanned skin can still suffer sunburn. A suntan only offers modest protection against further exposure.

Who is most at risk of UVR damage?

UVR damage occurs most easily in fair-skinned people and others who burn easily in the sun. Even dark-skinned people can get sunburnt. Everyone is at risk from UVR damage to the eyes.

How does UVR damage the eyes?

One-off intense exposure (as in snow blindness) can cause intense inflammation in the eye. High levels of exposure over a long time may

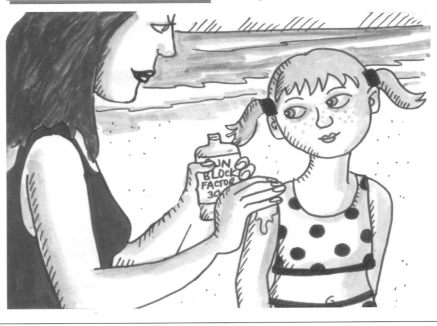

Family and friends

Information from Macmillan Cancer Relief

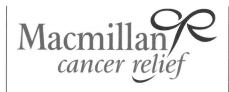

Family and friends provide vital support for a person with cancer. But they often feel uncertain about what to do, or feel they are not helping enough. There is much you can do, but no magic formula for what it should be. Everyone has different skills and capabilities. Listening, helping with practical tasks and finding out information can all be very valuable. But it is important not to try and do everything: you need to look after yourself too, so that you can be there when you are needed.

Listening and understanding

Usually, it's not what you say to a person with cancer which matters most to them, but how you listen.

Having cancer can give rise to a whole range of strong emotions: shock, fear, anger, bitterness, uncertainty, confusion, depression. All too easily people with cancer can feel vulnerable and isolated. Talking about fears can actually help reduce anxiety.

You can help by encouraging the person to talk, and by acknowledging the unpleasantness of all these feelings. Not all of us are born counsellors, but if you are a good listener, you can show a person with cancer that you accept how they feel. That might help them be more comfortable with talking openly.

Tips for good listening

Getting a conversation going is sometimes difficult. You might find the following tips useful:

- Give clues that you are not hurrying off: sit down, take your coat off
- Get on the same level as the person you are talking to, and not too far away
- If you're not sure whether the other person wants to talk, you can always ask. (Do you feel like talking?) Try not to be offended if the other person does not want to talk.

If the conversation does get under way, you can help the other person say what's on their mind by:

- Actually listening to what they are saying, rather than thinking about what you are going to say next
- Encouraging them, by saying things like 'yes' and 'I see' as they talk, or holding their hand if they are obviously thinking about something painful
- Showing you're listening by picking up on things they have said
- Being honest – and not afraid of describing your own feelings
- Allowing silences, and not filling them with words for the sake of it
- Not changing the subject, even if you find some of the things being said difficult
- Not interrupting, or blocking their flow by saying things like 'You'll be alright' or 'Don't worry'
- Not forcing your advice on the other person: try presenting your suggestions as questions, such as 'Have you ever thought about?'

Good communication is not always easy to achieve, but it is very important to most relationships. Tackling a crisis like cancer has been known to strengthen people's relationships because they talk about things they have never confronted before. Secrecy, on the other hand, can damage trust and lead to a breakdown of communication – even if it is used to protect people.

Giving practical help

Some people find it easier to give practical help than emotional support.

But it is often difficult to know where to start. Here are some suggestions:

1. Offer to help

If you are not one of the immediate family, find out if your help is needed.

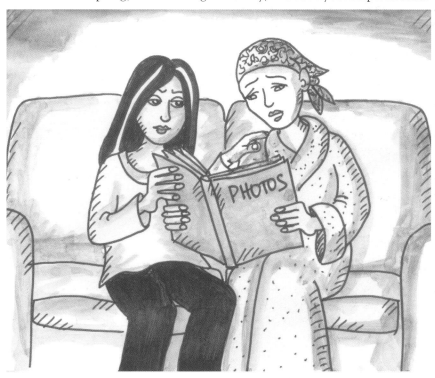

2. Assess what the person needs most

Ask yourself what they will be able to do for themselves during each day, and what they will not. For example, if the person is at home between chemotherapy sessions: 'Who is going to look after her in the day?'; 'Can she prepare her own meals?'; 'Do the children need to be taken to and from school?'

3. Decide which of these jobs you can do

For example, you may be working in the day, and you may be a terrible cook, but you have a car and could take the children to school in the morning.

4. Start with small practical things

From the list of things you can do, offer one or two. Remember that sometimes it is the small thoughtful offers that mean most: like offering to tend their garden. Large gifts can overwhelm and embarrass people.

5. You can always offer to visit

Spending regular time with your friend or relative, and being reliable about your visits, could be the most valuable way you can give practical help.

Becoming informed

Those close to a person with cancer will usually need to know about the medical situation if they are to have an idea of what will help. Doctors are usually happy to keep close relatives informed, as long as the person they are treating agrees.

Many family members, friends and carers find that the more they know about cancer and the help available, the better equipped they feel to cope. Cancer organisations and health professionals should all be aware that families and carers have

Those close to a person with cancer will usually need to know about the medical situation if they are to have an idea of what will help

information needs, and will help you find out what you need to know.

Sometimes the person with cancer finds it's useful for such information to be passed on to them. But you should wait to be asked, and not assume that they need the same sort of information as you do. People with cancer need to be encouraged to get through their treatment, not overwhelmed with conflicting advice. You should make sure that the information you provide is accurate and relevant to their situation.

Looking after yourself

The last thing a person with cancer needs is for those close to them to become ill. So family and friends have a responsibility to look after themselves.

That means being fair to yourself and recognising your own limitations. If you are realistic and practical, you can do a lot towards solving problems. If you attempt big gestures and fail, or become ill yourself in the

Tips for looking after yourself

- Keep your own health appointments, and tell your doctor if you are caring for someone with cancer
- Eat well – at least one proper meal a day
- If you feel unwell, get some extra rest and don't put off seeing your doctor
- Don't hesitate to turn to others for help
- Try and get a good night's sleep
- Try and keep up regular gentle exercise – it can be relaxing and give you more energy
- Try to make time for yourself every day
- Try and share your feelings – a local carers' group may help
- Try to keep your social life going if you can – at least by phoning people
- Try and recognise the signs of stress – do you have headaches, insomnia, digestive problems, constant colds?
- Try relaxation techniques: ask your family doctor for advice

process, you became part of the problem. So recognise what you cannot do, don't feel guilty about it, and get other people to help.

Most organisations for people with cancer provide support for close family and friends. Local branches, or self-help groups, are particularly suited to giving personalised help. Some health professionals, such as Macmillan nurses, specialise in offering support to the whole family from diagnosis onwards.

Sometimes talking to friends can be a help, but many organisations and local groups can also provide a listening ear

Using such 'outsiders' can provide you with:

- Information – being armed with facts, and having an idea of what to expect, can make some people feel better
- Practical, and possibly financial, help/advice
- Someone professional to talk to, who might help get things into perspective

Inevitably, close family and friends of people with cancer feel great strain, and they too should take care not to bottle up their feelings. Sometimes talking to friends can be a help, but many organisations and local groups can also provide a listening ear.

Family and close friends should try and keep physically healthy by getting plenty of rest and eating properly. Sometimes this isn't easy, particularly if you are looking after someone who needs a lot of care at home. But remember that there are organisations which can give you a break, or help with nursing.

- The above information is an extract from *The Cancer Guide*, produced by the BBC and Macmillan Cancer Relief. See page 41 for Macmillan's address details or visit their web site at www.macmillan.org.uk

© 2002 BBC/Macmillan Cancer Relief

You and your doctors

Information from Macmillan Cancer Relief

If you have cancer, you will come into contact with a whole range of health professionals who should work closely together to provide you with care and support. However, it is likely that doctors will be the first people to talk to you about your condition, and they will continue to be an important point of contact throughout your cancer journey.

Your family doctor

Your family doctor or GP (general practitioner) should co-ordinate the help you want throughout your treatment and beyond. They are responsible for all aspects of your medical care at home, and can arrange help from other professionals such as nurses.

They should:

- Answer your questions
- Talk to you about your cancer, its effects, and how to cope
- Discuss with you the options for treatment, what effects it might have and where it might take place
- Refer you to the clinic or hospital which offers the services you need
- As part of a team of professionals, organise services to help you live at home with the support you need to make the quality of life of you and your family as good as possible

Remember you can:

- Ask to be referred to a specialist who is acceptable to you
- Ask to see your medical records
- Talk to your GP if you are unhappy with any aspect of your care
- Change to another GP if, after talking to your current doctor, you continue to be unhappy with the way you are being treated. You may need to change your health centre to do so
- Make a complaint, if things do not improve. You can write to your Local Health Authority, or contact NHS Direct for advice.

Alternatively, you can contact your local Community Health Council (Local Health Councils in Scotland, Health and Social Services Councils in Northern Ireland) for guidance. You will find the number in your local phone book.

It can be difficult to take action and say what you want if you are feeling ill or uncertain. But remember it is all right to do so, and some of the organisations at the end of this article can help support you.

Your hospital doctor

Your family doctor will refer you to a hospital doctor or specialist (a doctor who specialises in a particular area of medicine). An oncologist is a cancer specialist, but not all cancer patients currently get to see this kind of doctor. You may wish to ask to be referred to an oncologist. You may also wish to be referred to a specialist for the part of the body where the cancer is located if surgery is involved.

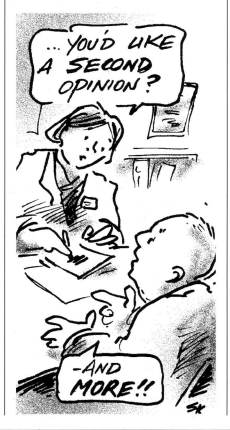

The most senior specialists are consultants, who supervise the work of a team of doctors, which might include grades such as house officer, senior house officer and specialist registrar.

Remember you can:

- Ask the doctor to explain any proposed treatment and its side-effects before you agree to it
- Ask to be referred to an oncologist
- Ask to be referred to a doctor who specialises in the part of the body where your cancer is located
- Ask for a second opinion. You can ask any of the doctors looking after you about this
- Talk to your doctors if you are unhappy with any aspect of your treatment. If you remain unhappy, you can discuss the matter with your Community Health Council (Local Health Councils in Scotland, Health and Social Services Councils in Northern Ireland) or ask NHS Direct for advice. You can also write to the chief executive or complaints officer of the hospital you are attending
- Take some time before making decisions, and consult the organisations listed at the end of this article to help you

Talking to your doctors

Doctors are busy people and their time is often limited. You may feel rushed when you are with them. But it is important that you ask for an explanation if you don't understand anything your doctor tells you. Even if the doctor is being very clear and thorough, it may be difficult to take in what is being said, particularly if you are worried. To help you remember the conversation, you could try:

- Bringing a friend or relative to consultations
- Making notes before, during and after your visit
- Using a tape-recorder. Check that the doctor has no objection first.

Questions to ask your doctors

Throughout the process of diagnosis and treatment, you will keep on thinking of things you want to know about – usually just after you have walked out of the doctor's office. It is sometimes useful to jot down some of the questions you want to ask before each visit. Your family doctor may not be able to answer all your questions because GPs are not cancer experts. But if they cannot help, you should be able to get an answer from your hospital doctor.

What follows are some questions patients commonly ask their GP and specialist. There are no right or wrong questions and no right time to ask them – you can ask any question at any time. But these might help jog your memory.

Questions when your family doctor refers you for tests

- What do you think is wrong with me?
- What tests will I need?
- Where will I go for the tests?
- When will I know the results?
- Who will explain what the results mean?
- Who will you refer me to for specialist treatment?
- What choices do I have about treatment?
- What difference will it make if I go privately?
- How much will it cost to go privately?

Questions when you see the hospital doctor

- What tests and treatments are there?
- What do the tests and treatments involve?
- Are there any other methods of treatment?
- Where will I have to go for treatment?
- What are the benefits of the different options for treatment?
- What choice do I have?
- What are the risks and side-effects of the treatments?
- Will they affect my work/education?
- How experienced are you and your team in the type of surgery proposed?
- What is your success rate with the surgery proposed?
- Will I need help to look after my family?
- Can I still have sex?
- Will treatment affect my chances of having children in the future?
- How can I tell my family and friends?
- How long will the treatment last?
- How do I know I'm getting the best treatment?
- Will my treatment affect driving?

In some families and relationships, the person with cancer and those close to them might have different viewpoints, and may want to ask their questions privately. This applies particularly to families where a child or young person has cancer.

Questions during treatment

- How can I tell if the treatment is working?

- What happens when the treatment finishes?
- What can I do to help myself?
- Is there anything I should avoid?
- Who can I talk to about what I should eat?

Questions after treatment

- When will I know if the treatment has worked?
- How long will it be before I feel better and can get back to my normal routine?
- What happens next?
- When do I next see you?
- What happens if the treatment hasn't worked?
- How will I know if the treatment has caused long-term damage?
- Who can provide help for me at home?
- Is there any financial help available for people like me?

Questions for the parent

- How can I make sure my daughter/son gets the best treatment and best support?
- Will my daughter/son be treated with older people or other young people?
- What should we tell our other children?
- Will our other children need help?
- Can I talk to other parents of young people with cancer?
- Where will my daughter/son be treated?

Questions for the young patient

- Do other people of my age get cancer?
- Can I talk to the doctor without my mum or dad?
- What sort of ward will I be in?
- Is there somewhere I can be treated with people of my own age?
- Can I still go out and continue at school/college?
- My mum and dad won't cope – what will I say to them?
- I'm frightened of what my friends will say. How can I handle that?
- Will I be able to live a normal life when I grow up?

Who to ask

- The Patients' Association
- The National Cancer Alliance publishes a *Directory of Cancer Specialists*
- NHS Direct
- Your local Community Health Council (Local Health Councils in Scotland, Health and Social Services Councils in Northern Ireland)
- Citizens' Advice Bureau or Health Authority (look in your phone book)

- The above information is an extract from *The Cancer Guide*, produced by the BBC and Macmillan Cancer Relief. See page 41 for Macmillan's address details or visit their web site at www.macmillan.org.uk

© 2002 BBC/Macmillan Cancer Relief

Fighting the big 'C'

A guide for young people (cancer patients) and their families to understanding cancer and its treatment. By Sister Sarah J. Palmer

What is cancer?

Our bodies are made up of millions and millions of cells.

There are about 200 different types of cells which all do different jobs, have different shapes, and behave in different ways: for example, a muscle cell is different from a bone cell, which is different to a skin cell etc. New cells are made to help us grow or repair old worn-out cells.

Some cells will carry on dividing throughout our lives in a special way so that new healthy cells are produced. However, if something goes wrong when they are dividing so that an abnormal cell is produced, this cell will divide again and again giving us more and more abnormal cells. These abnormal cells are the cancer cells.

Cancer cells tend to divide and grow quicker than normal cells. Cancer is the word given to an abnormal growth of cells in the body which is malignant.

Malignant means the abnormal cells are able to spread to other parts of the body if they are not treated.

There are two main types of cancer:
1. Solid cancers – when a lump forms, e.g. the bone, muscle, brain cells, etc. divide and multiply abnormally.
2. Leukaemias and lymphomas – when the blood cells divide and multiply abnormally.

There are a number of ways in which cancer can be treated:
- Chemotherapy
- Radiotherapy
- Surgery

The treatment the doctors choose for you depends on the type of cancer you have and the stage that it has reached. You may receive one treatment, a combination or all three of these different types of treatments. The doctors will decide on a special plan of treatment for you or protocol and will explain exactly what is going to happen.

Please remember that:
- you cannot catch cancer from anyone else
- you cannot give cancer to anyone if you have it
- nobody knows why some people develop cancer and others do not
- it is nothing you have done or said that has caused it

Did you know that cancers are not only found in people but in animals and plants as well?

What is chemotherapy?

The word 'chemotherapy' comes from two words: 'chemo' and 'therapy' meaning 'chemical' and 'treatment'.

Chemotherapy is the use of drugs (chemicals) to destroy the cancer cells.

These anti-cancer drugs are sometimes referred to as cytotoxic drugs.

Often you will need several different drugs to treat your type of cancer.

When the doctors have decided on your treatment plan (or protocol)

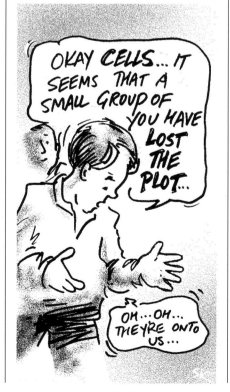

they will tell you about:
- Each type of drug and what it is called;
- Any side-effects;
- How often you will need it;
- How it will be given to you (as a tablet, medicine, injection, or as an infusion of the drug diluted in fluid and given into the vein, i.e. through a drip). Should you be undergoing treatment, please discuss your chemotherapy in more depth with your doctors and nurses.

What is radiotherapy?

The word 'radiotherapy' comes from two words: 'radio' and 'therapy' meaning 'radiation' and 'treatment'.

Radiotherapy is the use of radiation treatment or high energy rays which destroy the cancer cells, while doing as little harm as possible to normal cells. Radiotherapy is not painful and only lasts a few minutes. It is like having an x-ray taken. You will have to lie very still. Only some people will need this type of treatment, depending on the type of cancer they have.

Your doctor will tell you if you will be having radiotherapy and will discuss it in much more depth with you and any side-effects it may have.

What is surgery?

Surgery means to have an operation.

Operations are done in an operating theatre in hospital. You will have a general anaesthetic which will send you to sleep so that when you wake up the operation will be finished and you will not remember or know anything about having it. After your operation you will be given some pain-killers, but please tell the nurses if you are still uncomfortable and they will try to help you further.

If you have a lump or a tumour you may need to have a *BIOPSY* taken. A biopsy is when a small piece of the lump or tumour is removed. The doctors can then examine it under a microscope and do some special tests on it to find out more about it and therefore reach a diagnosis. This is done as a small operation.

The nurses and doctors will tell you a lot more about operations if you need to have one.

Your blood and bone marrow

Your blood is made up from three main types of blood cells:

- Red blood cells – carry oxygen around the body.
- White blood cells – fight infections.
- Platelets – help to clot the blood to prevent bleeding and bruising.

Blood is made in your bone marrow, which is a spongy material in the middle of your bones. Normally blood cells are produced constantly throughout your life.

All bones help to make new blood cells, although some make a lot more than others.

Our bone marrow is like a factory that is producing new cells all the time. The cells in your bone marrow divide rapidly to produce new blood cells.

The cells that divide rapidly in our body are affected by chemotherapy and radiotherapy in the following way:

Types of cells affected:	Effect of chemotherapy/ radiotherapy:
cancer cells	kills the cancer
blood cells	reduces the number of blood cells
hair cell	causes hair loss
cells in the mouth and gut	causes a sore mouth

Radiotherapy is usually given to a particular area of the body. For example, if you had a lump on your leg, only that area of your body would be treated and you would lose the hair on that part of your leg.

Chemotherapy affects the bone marrow of all the bones of the body and therefore the number of blood cells that are made.

If you receive chemotherapy the number of blood cells produced will get less or 'drop'. We say your 'blood count' has dropped, which is usually at its lowest point 10 days after the start of your treatment.

Red blood cells

Red blood cells are responsible for carrying oxygen around the body.

They contain an iron compound called haemoglobin (Hb) which helps to carry the oxygen.

A low number of red blood cells (a low Hb) is called 'anaemia'.

Someone with this condition is described as being 'anaemic'.

If you become anaemic because of your treatment you may:

- feel tired and lack energy
- look pale
- become breathless when doing only a little exercise
- feel the cold more than normal
- feel dizzy and have headaches

Your normal red blood cell count or Hb is between 12 and 14 (some hospitals measure this as 120 to 140, both are correct, just different units used). Your body can usually manage to make enough red blood cells again but if your Hb falls to as low as 8 (or 80) then you may be given a blood transfusion.

This is a bag (or unit) of blood given through a drip into your veins. This will be given in hospital over several hours, about 3 to 4 hours per unit of blood.

White blood cells

White blood cells are the main fighting cells in our blood.

They help fight off infections that come from bacteria, viruses or fungal agents.

When there is a low number of white blood cells in our blood we can develop infections much more easily than normal.

There are three main types of white blood cells:

- Neutrophils [also called granulocytes or polymorphs (polys)]
- Lymphocytes
- Monocytes

Together they make up the total white blood count – normally 4 to 10. (Which is actually 4,000 to 10,000 white blood cells per cubic millimetre of blood!)

The cells we are particularly concerned with are the neutrophils. The normal neutrophil count is between 2 and 6.

When a sample of your blood is taken and checked and the neutrophil count is less than 1 we say you are neutropenic. A low number of neutrophils is called neutropenia.

You will have to wait for the body to make its own white cells again in the bone marrow 'factory' as we do not give white blood cells as a transfusion.

Platelets

Platelets are tiny cells which help to clot the blood to prevent bleeding and bruising.

A low number of platelets is called 'thrombocytopenia'. If your platelets are low it is said you are 'thrombocytopenic'.

You may:

- bruise more easily
- bleed for longer than normal if you cut yourself
- have nosebleeds
- have bleeding gums
- develop pin-prick bruises called 'petechiae'
- find that your urine or stools change colour, due to traces of blood.
- have headaches

Your normal platelet count is between 150 and 400. (Which is actually 150,000 to 400,000 per cubic millimetre of blood!)

If your platelet count falls to about 20 you may require a platelet transfusion.

This will be given in hospital and usually takes about half an hour depending on how many units of platelets need to be transfused.

Never take aspirin or tablets containing aspirin as they affect the blood clotting – it thins the blood making the time for the blood to clot even longer and you will bruise more easily. 'Bonjela' and 'Teejel' used to relieve the discomfort of a sore mouth and/or ulcers also contain aspirin, so please do not use these either. You may use 'Calgel', this is a paracetamol/calpol based gel which can help relieve localised pain from mouth sores.

■ The above information is from CLIC – Cancer and Leukaemia in Childhood's web site which can be found at www.clic.uk.com

© CLIC – Cancer and Leukaemia in Childhood

Controlling cancer

Information from www.schoolscience.org.uk

Surgery

A surgeon may be able to remove a tumour by cutting it out. For some types of cancer, surgery offers the best chance of cure – for example in treating cancer of the testis or ovary where a single tumour might develop.

Laser treatment is sometimes used to remove abnormal cells in the very early stage of development, before cancer can take hold.

Treatment with medicines

Chemotherapy is a treatment that involves using chemicals. Many different substances are used. Although they work in different ways, the result is the same – they all block cell division. They target fast-growing cells which include cancer cells but also healthy hair follicle cells. This is why people on chemotherapy often lose their hair.

Chemotherapy may be the only treatment someone needs. But medicines may also be used after a tumour has been removed by surgery. This is to ensure that any cells that have not been removed with the tumour are killed by the medicine. Sometimes chemotherapy is combined with radiotherapy.

Hormone treatment can also be used – for example in cases of breast cancer or prostate cancer. These cancers need the body's hormones in order to grow. By reducing the body's production of the necessary hormone, the cancer's growth is halted.

Bone marrow transplants can be used to treat leukaemia. Most types of leukaemia cause abnormal white blood cells to be produced by the bone marrow. A transplant of bone marrow from a suitable donor results in production of normal white cells to help the body fight infection and other diseases.

Vaccines are being tested to see if they can stimulate the body's own defences – the immune system – to destroy cancer cells.

Drugs to reduce the blood supply to a tumour are being tested. It is

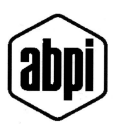

hoped that they will cause tumour cells to die by shutting off the cells' supply of oxygen and nutrients.

Other types of drugs such as epidermal growth factor receptor blockers are also being tested. These

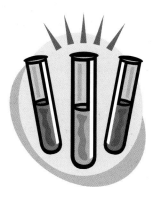

prevent receptors on cells from receiving the signals that make the cell divide.

Radiotherapy

Radiotherapy uses ionising radiation, usually gamma rays, to treat cancer. The main effect of radiation is to kill rapidly dividing cells. Since some healthy cells also divide rapidly, the gamma rays are aimed very carefully at the tumour.

Choosing an isotope

The radioactive isotope cobalt-60 is often used as a source of gamma rays, which are directed at the tumour.

Sometimes a radioactive isotope is used because it will be absorbed by the organ or tissue concerned. For example:
- a radioactive isotope of phosphorus is used to treat bone cancer, because bone contains a lot of phosphorus
- a radioactive isotope of iodine is

used to treat thyroid cancer because the iodine will be taken up by the thyroid gland to produce hormones such as thyroxin.

Radioactive materials or medicines may in future be attached to antibodies which target cancer cells. It is hoped that this approach might reduce the number of healthy cells harmed by these treatments.

Body scanning

Many people do survive cancer. What's more, the chances of surviving are improving all the time.

The sooner that cancer is detected, the greater the chance there is of a cure.

Advances in medical science mean that cancer can be detected earlier and that better treatments are available. For example, body scanners are important pieces of medical technology. They can detect where a tumour is very accurately.

Treatment and survival

Many thousands of new cancer cases occur each year.

The choice of treatment depends on the type of cancer, where it is and how far it has developed. Treatments include surgery, the use of anti-cancer medicines (chemotherapy) and radiotherapy, or a combination of these.

Many thousands of new cancer cases occur each year. The choice of treatment depends on the type of cancer, where it is and how far it has developed

---

■ The above information is from the schoolscience web site which can be found at www.schoolscience.co.uk
© The Association of the British Pharmaceutical Industry (ABPI)

The right to know

A CancerBACUP guide to information and support for people living with cancer

Introduction

There is a clear need to set standards of information and support for people with cancer, their families and friends. CancerBACUP, the leading national cancer information, counselling and support charity, has been working with more than 50 relevant organisations to begin to identify good practice in this area for people affected by cancer.

CancerBACUP brought together people with cancer, health professionals and representatives from the professional and voluntary organisations involved in their care. This article outlines the guiding principles identified by that group. It is hoped that these principles will form the basis for standards that health providers and others may set for themselves. Further, that people affected by cancer anywhere in the country will be able to receive the high quality information, counselling and support they need.

The need for improved information and support is well documented[1] and emphasised in the Calman report, which recommended: 'patients, families and carers should be given clear information and assistance in a form they can understand about treatment options and outcomes available to them at all stages of treatment from diagnosis onwards'.[2]

People who use CancerBACUP's services confirm that doctors, nurses and hospital staff often do not have the time to discuss in detail information about their disease or its emotional impact.

CancerBACUP supports the view that adequate resources and staff dedicated and trained for the task are essential to meet the information, counselling and support needs of people with cancer.

In the last year alone, Cancer-BACUP has helped people with cancer and their families through:
- 34,000 calls and letters answered by our specialist cancer information service nurses;
- 2,400 face-to-face sessions with our professional counsellors;
- a total of 200,000 copies of our 46 booklets on cancer, its treatment and living with cancer.

Effects of a diagnosis of cancer

There are one million people living with cancer: 1 in 3 people will develop cancer at some stage during their lifetime.[3]

Any diagnosis of cancer profoundly changes a person's life. People with cancer, their families and friends are likely to experience panic, despair and uncertainty. This will affect every aspect of their lives, especially their relationships and how they perceive their situation and their future

People with cancer leave a familiar and secure world and enter a new one of hospitals, specialists, medical terminology, medications and treatments. Up to the time of diagnosis, the only doctor most people may have encountered is the GP at the surgery, whom they may have known for years. Now, however, they may be referred to a range of specialists at an unfamiliar cancer hospital, who may advise on a variety of frightening treatment options.

Faced with such difficulties and new circumstances, people with cancer are frequently not given enough information to enable them to understand their illness, treatment options and side-effects – or even which specialist to call if there is an emergency. The diagnosis is likely to be given by a specialist who can spend only a few minutes in discussion. In most cases it is left to the patient to seek out resources to help him or her understand and come to terms with the illness at a time when this may be extremely difficult.

The need for improved information and support is well documented

---

Vital support

Everyone affected by a diagnosis of cancer should have access to a range of information and emotional and social support tailored to their own particular needs. Relevant, up-to-date information and appropriate support will improve understanding and help people manage their cancer and its treatment. This should include all aspects of treatment and recognise the particular physical, psychological, spiritual, social and emotional needs that a diagnosis of cancer brings.

Information and support to people with cancer will improve the quality of their lives and reduce uncertainty, anxiety and depression.[4]

It will also increase their satisfaction with the services they receive, their sense of involvement in their treatment, and communication between people with cancer, their families and friends and the staff involved in their care. It will thereby improve the effectiveness of the care they receive.[5]

References

1 *What Seems To Be The Matter: Communications Between Hospitals And Patients.* Audit Commission 1993 HMSO, London.
2 *A Policy Framework For Commissioning Cancer Services. Expert Advisory Group On Cancer To The Chief Medical Officer* (The Calman Report) 1995. Department Of Health, London.
3 Factsheet 1.1: *Incidence: UK Cancer Research Campaign.* 1994.
4 Ley, Philip. *Towards Better Doctor-Patient Communications.* In Jennet A E (ed).
5 *Communication Between Doctors And Patients.* 1976 Oxford University Press.

Complementary approaches

Information from Macmillan Cancer Relief

There are dozens of different types of complementary therapies. By choosing a complementary therapy to suit their particular needs, many people with cancer feel they regain some genuine control over their own health.

Practitioners of complementary care usually take a holistic approach, which means you are seen as a whole person, with your body, mind and spirit all inter-related and contributing to your state of health. Rather than treating just one part of your body, it is likely that a complementary practitioner will want to know about how you feel in a broader sense.

Complementary therapists try to support cancer patients through their treatment and after. Some people have found that complementary therapies have helped reduce the side-effects of their treatment. By focusing closely on your emotional and psychological well-being, they can also reduce stress.

Although some of the complementary approaches are available through the NHS and many doctors think they can be very useful, they are not always accepted by the medical establishment. This is partly because, until recently, they have not been subject to the strict medical trials by which doctors prove a treatment works. On the other hand, very many people who have had cancer say they have felt real benefits from using them.

If you decide to start using complementary therapy, it is wise to tell your doctor, who will probably be quite supportive of your decision.

> *Some people with cancer have decided to take complementary care instead of, rather than alongside, conventional medical care*

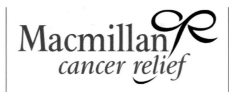

Types of complementary therapies

- Acupuncture
- Alexander technique
- Aromatherapy
- Art therapy
- Healing
- Herbalism
- Homoeopathy
- Massage
- Meditation
- Reflexology
- Relaxation
- Shiatsu
- Visualisation
- Yoga

If not, it might be an idea to ask if they have valid medical reasons against your choice.

Some people with cancer have decided to take complementary care instead of, rather than alongside, conventional medical care. This is not a decision that doctors are likely to view enthusiastically unless they feel that conventional treatment is no longer appropriate. Before taking this course of action, it is important to discuss it carefully with those close to you, your doctors, complementary practitioners and cancer support groups.

Dos and don'ts checklist for complementary therapy

Do
- Find a reliable practitioner. Recommendations are useful, but it is also worth checking whether there is an organisation that sets standards in the field, and if they have a list of qualified practitioners
- Try and find someone who has worked with people with cancer

- Check on the cost. Most therapies are not available on the NHS and can be expensive. It is worth checking what the cost of treatments should be with a recognised organisation for the therapy you choose
- Check the number of sessions needed before benefits are felt, and how long each session will take
- Choose someone you feel comfortable with

Don't
- Be afraid to ask for credentials and references
- Be led to believe there are 'miracle cures'
- Be taken in by people who say you should follow their method and abandon everything else

For more information
Who to ask
- The Institute for Complementary Medicine Tel: 020 7237 5165
- The Foundation for Integrated Medicine Tel: 020 7688 1881
- The Bristol Cancer Help Centre Tel: 0117 980 9500
- National Federation of Spiritual Healers, Old Manor Farm Studio, Church Street, Sunbury on Thames TW16 6RG Tel: 01932 783164
- British Acupuncture Council Tel: 020 8735 0400
- British Homeopathic Association, 27a Devonshire Street, London W1N 1RJ Tel: 020 7935 2163
- Cancerlink (now part of Macmillan Cancer Relief) publishes a booklet on *Complementary Care and Cancer*.

- The above information is an extract from *The Cancer Guide*, produced by the BBC and Macmillan Cancer Relief. See page 41 for Macmillan's address details or visit their web site at www.macmillan.org.uk

- There are around 200 different types of cancer, depending on the cell type involved, and they vary greatly from each other and in the types of treatment needed. (p. 01)

- More than 70 per cent of cancers are preventable. (p.01)

- Cancer has become the main cause of death in both men and women. Between 1950 and 1999, deaths due to cancer rose from 15 to 27 per cent in men and from 16 to 23 per cent in women – overtaking heart disease, stroke and infectious diseases as the other major killers in England and Wales. (p. 02)

- There are over 200 different types of cancer but the four major types, lung, breast, prostate and colorectal, account for over half of all cases diagnosed. (P. 03)

- In the case of the first stage of breast cancer, five-year survival in the UK was 78%, compared with 97% in the US and 93% in other EU countries. (p. 06)

- Children's cancers are rare. Only 1 in every 600 children under 15 years of age develops a cancer. (p. 08)

- Cancers are not infectious, nor, for most cancers, is there any evidence that they are inherited. (p. 08)

- Leukaemia is the most common type of childhood cancer, representing about one-third of all cancers in under-15-year-olds. (p. 09)

- In the UK around , 1,450 children receive a diagnosis of cancer each year and the majority of these children will be successfully treated. There are now over 13,000 adult survivors of childhood cancer in the UK and the evidence is that they are virtually indistinguishable from their peers. (p. 10)

- Three-quarters of children say that they would like to know more about cancer. (p. 12)

- One in four people in England will die of cancer. More than one in three people will develop cancer at some stage in their lives. (p. 13)

- Mortality rates for breast cancer have fallen by over 20% over the past decade (p. 13)

- Falls in the rate of smoking among men since the early 1970s have led to a marked fall in the incidence and death rate from lung cancer. (p. 13)

- Overall, the number of people surviving more than five years has improved – an average of 4% every five years. (p. 13)

- One in two smokers dies prematurely: of these, nearly one in four will die of lung cancer. (p. 15)

- Although 90% of the world's 1.2 million cases of lung cancer every year are caused by smoking, tobacco is now thought to increase the risk of developing many other kinds of cancer as well. (p. 17)

- Deaths from the worst form of skin cancer have more than trebled over the past 40 years because people are oblivious to the dangers. (p. 19)

- 'In Scotland, new cases of melanoma have quadrupled since the 1960s, and there has been a similar increase in England and Wales.' (p. 19)

- 70-80% of patients with early cancer survive for more than 10 years after treatment. (p. 24)

- Prostate cancer will overtake lung cancer to become the most common form of the disease in men within four years. (p. 25)

- The disease affects around 22,000 men in Britain each year, and kills 10,000. (p. 25)

- There has been a 84% rise in incidence of testicular cancer in Britain since the late 1970s. The causes of this rise are unknown (p. 26)

- Death rates for the four biggest cancers in the UK – lung, breast, intestine and stomach – are all declining. (p. 27)

- Overall, around 70% of all childhood cancers are now successfully treated compared to less than 30% in the 1960s and for certain cancers the outlook is even better. (p. 28)

- Chemotherapy is the use of drugs (chemicals) to destroy the cancer cells. (p. 33)

- Radiotherapy is the use of radiation treatment or high energy rays which destroy the cancer cells, while doing as little harm as possible to normal cells. (p. 33)

- Some people with cancer have decided to take complementary care instead of, rather than alongside, conventional medical care. (p. 39)

You might like to contact the following organisations for further information. Due to the increasing cost of postage, many organisations cannot respond to enquiries unless they receive a stamped, addressed envelope.

ASH – Action on Smoking and Health
102 Clifton Street
London, EC2A 4HW
Tel: 020 7739 5902
Fax: 020 7613 0531
E-mail:
action.smoking.health@dial.pipex.com
Web site: www.ash.org.uk
ASH is working to secure public, media, parliamentary, local and national Government support for a comprehensive programme to tackle the epidemic of tobacco-related disease.

Breast Cancer Campaign
Clifton Centre
110 Clifton Street
London, EC2A 4HT
Tel: 020 7749 3700
Fax: 020 7749 3701
E-mail: info@bcc-uk.org
Web site: www.bcc-uk.org
The Breast Cancer Campaign is the only charity that specialises in funding independent breast cancer research throughout the United Kingdom.

Breast Cancer Care
Kiln House
210 New Kings Road
London, SW6 4NZ
Tel: 020 7384 2984
Fax: 020 7384 3387
Helpline: 0808 800 6000
Textphone: 0808 800 6001
E-mail: info@breastcancercare.org.uk
Web site: www.breastcancercare.org.uk
Breast Cancer Care is the leading provider of breast cancer information and support in the UK.

Cancer Research UK
PO Box 123
Lincoln's Inn Fields
London, WC2A 3PX
Tel: 020 7242 0200
Fax: 020 7269 3262
E-mail: publications@cancer.org.uk
Web site: www.cancerresearchuk.org
Cancer Research UK works to conquer cancer through world-class research. Runs CancerHelp UK (www.cancerhelp.org.uk) which is a free information service about cancer and cancer care for people with cancer and families.

CancerBACUP
3 Bath Place
Rivington Street
London, EC2A 3JR
Tel: 020 7696 9003
Fax: 020 7696 9002
Freephone helpline: 0808 800 1234
Web site: www.cancerbacup.org.uk
CancerBACUP's vision is to give cancer patients and their families the up-to-date information, practical advice and support they need to reduce the fear and uncertainty of cancer.

CLIC – Cancer and Leukaemia in Childhood
Abbey Wood
Bristol, BS34 7JU
Tel: 0117 311 2600
Fax: 0117 311 2649
E-mail: clic@clic-charity.demon.co.uk
Web site: www.clic.uk.com
CLIC's vision is of a world where cancer and leukaemia no longer threaten the lives of children.

Macmillan Cancer Relief
89 Albert Embankment
London, SE1 7UQ
Tel: 020 7840 7840
Fax: 020 7840 7841
CancerLine: 0808 808 2020
E-mail:
information_line@macmillan.org.uk
Web site: www.macmillan.org.uk
Macmillan Cancer Relief is a UK charity supporting people with cancer and their families with specialist information, treatment and care.

Marie Curie Cancer Care
89 Albert Embankment
London, SE1 7TP
Tel: 020 7599 7777
Fax: 020 7599 7788
E-mail: info@mariecurie.org.uk
Web site: www.mariecurie.org.uk
Marie Curie Cancer Care is dedicated to the care of people affected by cancer and the enhancement of their quality of like through its caring services, research and education.

National Radiological Protection Board (NRPB)
Chilton, Didcot, OX11 0RQ
Tel: 01235 831600
Fax: 01235 833891
E-mail: nrpb@nrpb.org
Web site: www.nrpb.org
NRPB works to advance the acquisition of knowledge about the protection of mankind from radiation hazards.

The Orchid Cancer Appeal
St Bartholomew's Hospital
London, EC1A 7BE
Tel: 020 7601 7808
Fax: 020 7796 0432
E-mail: info@orchid-cancer.org.uk
Web site: www.orchid-cancer.org.uk
The Orchid Cancer Appeal funds research into diagnosis, prevention and treatment of prostate and testicular cancer.

The Royal College of Radiologists
38 Portland Place
London, W1B 1JQ
Tel: 020 7636 4432
Fax: 020 7323 3100
E-mail: enquiries@rcr.ac.uk
Web site: www.rcr.ac.uk
The Royal College of Radiologists benefits patients, by encouraging the highest standards in the medical specialties of Clinical Radiology and Clinical Oncology.

Sargent Cancer Care for Children
Griffin House
161 Hammersmith Road
London, W6 8SG
Tel: 020 8752 2800
Fax: 020 8752 2806
E-mail: care@sargent.org
Web site: www.sargent.org
Each year over 2,000 children and young people under 21 are diagnosed with cancer. Sargent Cancer Care for Children supports families at home and in hospital from the day of diagnosis.

ACKNOWLEDGEMENTS

The publisher is grateful for permission to reproduce the following material.

While every care has been taken to trace and acknowledge copyright, the publisher tenders its apology for any accidental infringement or where copyright has proved untraceable. The publisher would be pleased to come to a suitable arrangement in any such case with the rightful owner.

Chapter One: Cancer

Cancer, © Marie Curie Cancer Care, Cancer is biggest killer, © Crown copyright is reproduced with the permission of Her Majesty's Stationery Office, Cancer statistics, © Cancer Research UK, The ten most common causes of death from cancer, © Cancer Research UK, The 20 most common cancers, © The Daily Mail, March 2002, UK cancer survival rates 'worst in Europe', © Guardian Newspapers Limited 2002, Cancer survival, © Crown copyright is reproduced with the permission of Her Majesty's Stationery Office, Common cancer myths, © CancerBACUP, Children's cancers, © CancerBACUP, Childhood cancer, © CancerBACUP, Childhood cancer, © Cancer Index, Children's tumours, © CancerBACUP, New cases of childhood cancer in the UK, © Cancer Research UK, Young people are confused and want to know more, © 2002 MORI, The challenge of cancer, © Crown copyright is reproduced with the permission of Her Majesty's Stationery Office, Cancer incidence, © Cancer Research UK, Cancer survival in the early 1990s: England and Wales lag behind, © Crown copyright is reproduced with the permission of Her Majesty's Stationery Office, Smoking and cancer, © ASH, WHO links passive smoking to cancers, © Guardian Newspapers Limited London 2002, Incident rates of lung cancer, © Crown copyright is reproduced with the permission of Her Majesty's Stationery Office, Body awareness, © Cancer Research UK, Skin cancer deaths soaring as we soak up the sun, © The Daily Mail, February 2002, Sunsense, © National Radiological Protection Board 2002, Breast health, © Breast Cancer Care, Age and breast cancer, © Breast Cancer Campaign, Risk of breast cancer, © Breast Cancer Campaign, Prostate cancer awareness, © The Orchid Cancer Appeal, Prostate cancer 'most common form by 2006', © Telegraph Group Limited, London 2002, Rates of prostate cancer, © Cancer Research UK, Testicular cancer awareness, © The Orchid Cancer Appeal, Testicular cancer, © Cancer Research UK.

Chapter Two: Fighting Cancer

UK leads way in reducing cancer toll, © Guardian Newspapers Limited London 2002, A friend in need, © Sargent Cancer Care for Children, Survival, © Cancer Research UK, Family and friends, © 2002 BBC/Macmillan Cancer Relief, You and your doctors, © 2002 BBC/Macmillan Cancer Relief, Fighting the big 'C', © CLIC – Cancer and Leukaemia in Childhood, Controlling cancer, © The Association of the British Pharmaceutical Industry (ABPI), Radiology, © The Royal College of Radiologists 2002, Wait for care, © Guardian Newspapers Limited London 2002, The right to know, © CancerBACUP, Complementary approaches, © 2002 BBC/Macmillan Cancer Relief.

Photographs and illustrations:

Pages 1, 19, 36: Pumpkin House; pages 7, 12, 15, 27, 31, 33: Simon Kneebone; pages 9, 20, 29: Bev Aisbett.

Craig Donnellan
Cambridge
January, 2003